D0373951

This book is dedicated to you, your brother, your dad, your boyfriend, your grandpa, your teacher, your mate, your homie, your BOYS and any guy ready to step into a more mindful way of living.

Now is the time to begin.

A guide to modern yoga and
living mindfully in the real world

SIT
DOWN

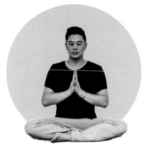

BE
QUIET

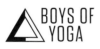
BOYS OF
YOGA

Thorsons

Michael James Wong

Foreword

To my son, and all the boys out there.

When you were younger you were a joy to be around. As you got older there were times your mother and I thought otherwise. But it didn't mean we ever stopped loving you. You were just growing up and figuring out who you wanted to be.

In the years that followed you were eager to learn more: about yourself, your family, your home, your community and how life worked when you had a little more time to experience it. There were good times, and times that didn't go exactly to plan. And that's ok, it's how life is supposed to be.

Parenting in any form is not an easy job and, like life, there is no roadmap. But I think we did alright. Our approach was simple; we encouraged you to have an open mind and a big heart and to understand that the world is a far nicer place when it's greeted with a hug or a high five. As your parents, we showed you life through the lens of our family, but allowed you the freedom to choose how you wanted to live and who you wanted to become.

We raised you to know that you are always more than enough.

We are from a different generation, and our greatest fear was that you would end up too much like us – outdated, behind the times and with an unwillingness to learn and grow with the ever-changing world.

Always remember to take risks, tell people you love them and say it like you mean it. You've only got one shot at this thing called life – make sure you live it to the fullest.

My wish is that this book opens the minds of more men of all ages to take to the mat, to become yogis of the future, for their own good and wellbeing. Since you started yoga, I've learned that it's not a casual pastime and it's not just something to make you more flexible, or calm your temper; it's the full package – a lifestyle and a wonderful, fulfilling and healthy way of living.

It's something I wish I had known more about when I was younger and I'm sure your mother would agree.

I'm extremely inspired by what you do, who you have become and your willingness to always stay true to your intentions. Never compromise on the things that make you happy, just keep smiling and enjoy the ride.

Lots of love
Dad

P.S. Don't forget to call your mum.

(Graham C. Wong, Santa Monica, California)

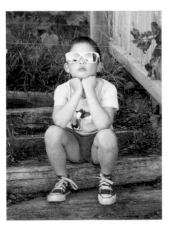

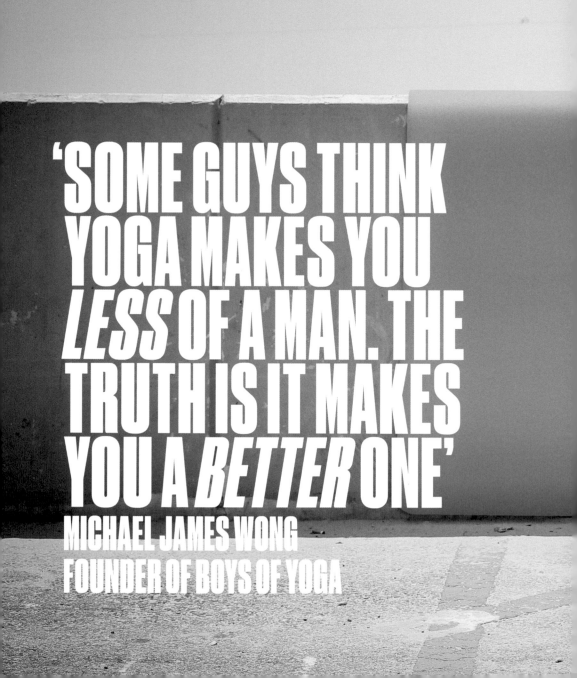
'SOME GUYS THINK YOGA MAKES YOU *LESS* OF A MAN. THE TRUTH IS IT MAKES YOU A *BETTER* ONE'

MICHAEL JAMES WONG
FOUNDER OF BOYS OF YOGA

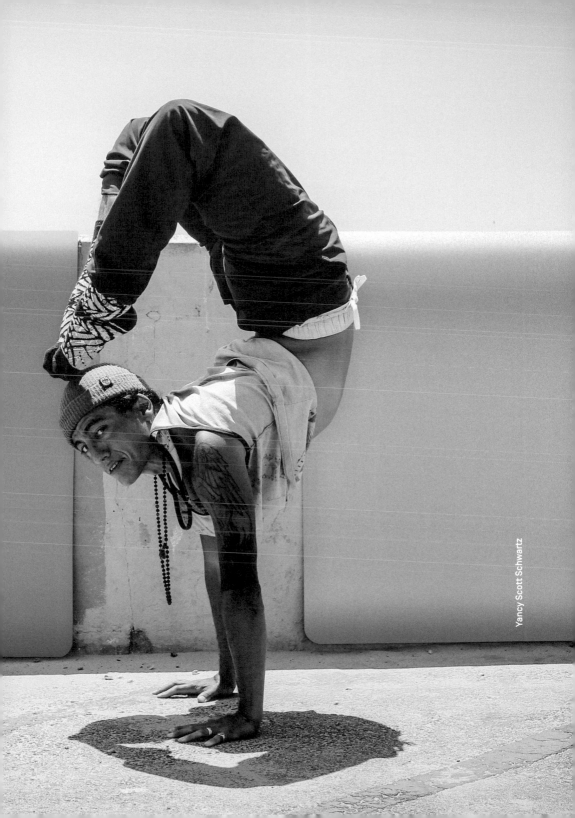

About Boys Of Yoga

To most guys yoga is pink Lycra and vegan chicks. It's breathing deeply while doing poses named after animals and feelings. It's done in dimly lit rooms with candles and incense, followed by gluten-free cupcakes and kale smoothies. And if that's your mentality, then you're not alone.

But it doesn't mean you're right. The real practice of yoga is working in, not working out. There is a lot more to it than just making shapes on the mat, and over time the body will get stronger and more flexible, the mind calmer and daily life will feel a little less chaotic. Yoga can give you the physical workout you want, but go deeper and you'll realise it's so much more.

'SMASH THE STEREOTYPE AND GET MORE GUYS ON THE MAT'

Unfortunately, these days the perception is still one-dimensional. Magazine pages and Instagram feeds are flooded with bikini-clad girls on the beach in all kinds of acrobatic poses reminiscent of the circus. Is this yoga? Yes, but it's not the full picture. Take one step back and widen your perspective and you'll see there is a whole other breed of yogi out there, the BOYS, inspiring, teaching and living yoga in their communities all around the world.

This is BOYS OF YOGA, the uncelebrated minority. A project aimed at sharing a different side of the yoga community in an authentic and unfiltered way.

What started as a casual conversation about guys being under-represented in the modern yoga community has turned into a movement to challenge the way we view and practise yoga in the Western world today.

The aim is simple: smash the stereotypes of yoga for guys and share the benefits that the practice offers both on and off the mat.

With inspiring stories and experiences shared by male yogis from around the world, this is a movement to change the world for the better. It's pretty simple: yoga is good for everyone and the benefits are undeniable.

Now is the time to get involved.

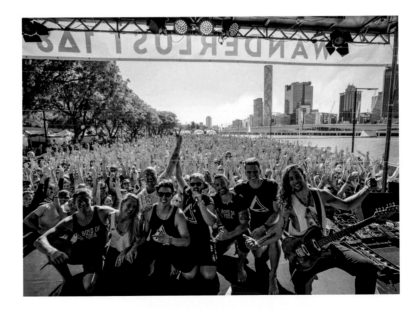

Find out more at boysofyoga.com @boysofyoga

Introduction

Hi, I'm Michael James Wong. Global Yogi, Wellness Warrior and founder of BOYS OF YOGA.

But before all of this, I was just a boy who was born in New Zealand and grew up on the beaches of Santa Monica, California. I was from a place no one had heard of until the *Lord of the Rings* movies and, growing up as an immigrant, I just wanted to fit in and belong.

In those days most of the other kids thought New Zealand and Madagascar were the same country (remember, this was before wifi and Facebook). On a good day, they assumed New Zealand was part of Australia. Growing up in LA, some kids looked at me as if I was from a distant planet and teased me because I had a 'resident alien' card in my wallet that my mom made me carry around to prove I was allowed to live in the US.

At the time, I lacked confidence and identity. I wasn't American (I didn't get my citizenship until I was 16) and I didn't feel Kiwi (I didn't have the accent and only visited once a year during the holidays). I'm also Chinese-Asian, something that I battled with growing up because it made life more confusing. I had the surname, but no ties to the culture or country other than weekend dinners and select colloquialisms. I was a bit from everywhere, and at the time I felt like I didn't belong anywhere. As a kid that was tough. But looking back I can see that it made me who I am today, and has allowed me to live the life I have now. And for that I'm forever grateful.

I had a pretty typical childhood in a liberal progressive city ... playing sports, being the drummer in a band, becoming a Boy Scout and living life in shorts and a t-shirt. I'm lucky to have an amazing family with supportive parents who have always been there for me, no matter what. My parents moved us to LA early in the 1980s because of work (my dad was the general manager of Canterbury of New Zealand back then) and in those early days when we had just moved to town I didn't have a lot of friends, so family life was everything.

My dad coached soccer and he never missed a game or school function and to this day is still a pillar in the Santa Monica social and sports community. My mom is the family rock – kind, thoughtful and compassionate. She taught me how to cook, be a gentleman, respect everyone and see the good in people. I don't think she has ever taken a night off, she really is the best mom in the world (in my humble opinion).

I am the middle child of three. I have an older brother, Andrew; he was the guy you always wanted on your side, not because he was a tough guy (though he frequently reminded me growing up who was in charge), but because he's loyal, trustworthy, honest and kind. I give a lot of credit to him for me turning out an ok human being. My little sister, Nicole, is the family superstar; straight-A student, artist, creative and Daddy's little princess. Even to this day she still puts her older brothers to shame and we expect nothing less.

After high school, I went to the University of California, Los Angeles (UCLA) on a music scholarship, but later gave it up and instead graduated with a degree in Sociology and the study of human behaviour. It was clear even back then that I enjoyed immersing myself in the study of real life, rather than notes on a page.

My journey with yoga started around 2005 and it changed my life for ever. Despite growing up in LA, yoga wasn't part of my vocabulary until my early 20s. When I started, I started reluctantly. A few friends dragged me to that first class and it felt awkward and intimidating. I just wasn't any good at yoga, and the problem was I thought I was supposed to be. Touching my toes is an ability that comes and goes daily and I'm certain my foot will never reach behind my head, but that's not really the point. Yoga has always been great to keep me fit and flexible, but the benefits are far greater than just this. Yoga changed, and saved, my life.

'YOGA CLEANSED ME, SHAPED ME AND GAVE ME SOMETHING TO BE INSPIRED BY'

Yoga gave me passion and perspective, something I'd never had growing up. I lived in a bubble; parties, late nights, all the glitzy superficiality that comes with growing up in LA. My reality was skewed and my ego over-inflated. I can honestly say I'm not sure how I would have turned out if I hadn't stumbled into that first class at City Yoga on Fairfax Avenue.

Yoga cleansed me, shaped me and gave me something to be inspired by. The asana (the physical practice) committed me to a daily dose of strength, flexibility and mobility; it gave me a challenge that I couldn't talk my way out of. These days, this part of the practice reminds me how lucky

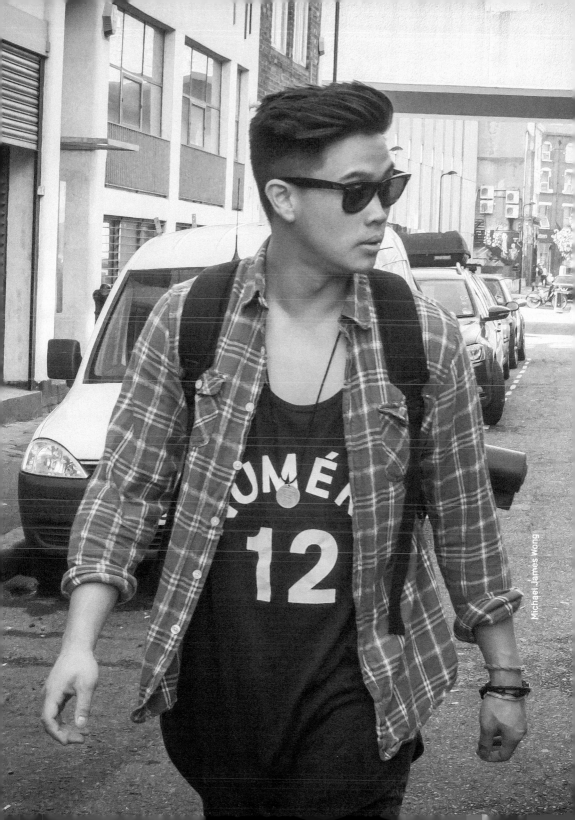

I am to be able to tie my own shoes, pick up and play with my niece, Koa, and walk away from things that don't serve my life.

Yoga gave me peace in a way I didn't even know I needed, the kind that helped me battle my daily insecurities. Even more, yoga helped to calm the chaos in my mind, manage my personal anxiety and perceive the world from a kinder point of view, one day at a time.

Through the practice, I've started to slow down. I'm quieter now than I used to be. I enjoy the silence. Beyond anything else, yoga has given me space, something I never knew was lacking in my life. Yoga helped me to find confidence in myself on and off the mat. Those first few years of dedicated practice allowed me to realise that life wasn't all about being cool.

'YOGA HELPED TO CALM THE CHAOS IN MY MIND'

At the age of 25 I left the US to travel the world and experience a little more of what life had to offer (to the anguish of my mother, I've yet to move back home). Since leaving, I've split my time between Sydney and London, getting my passport stamped in as many places as possible on the way.

And I'm still going. I've been teaching yoga, modern mindfulness and meditation for the past ten years and I am blessed to have an amazing community of yogis, teachers, students and friends all over the world.

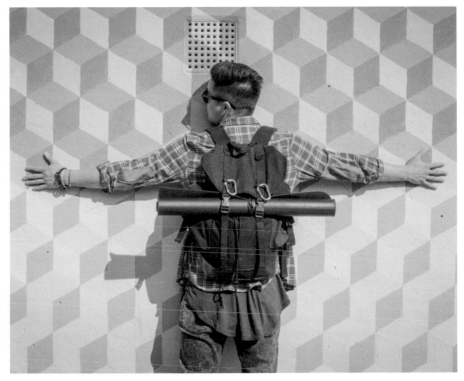

Michael James Wong

I give credit to my parents for my diverse upbringing and the trust and freedom they allowed me to continue exploring the world.

I'm grateful for all the choices I have made to get me to this point in my life. I always thank my parents for showing me the world through their eyes. I've been lucky enough to be an immigrant my whole life. I was raised to respect everyone from everywhere, because I was welcomed everywhere. Home has always been where friends and family are, and these days, no matter where I go I'm home.

This is me living my Yoga.

The Beginning

BOYS OF YOGA is a project inspired by the global community that exists and thrives all over the world.

The aim is to share and connect with male yogis around the world to help widen the common perception of the practice, and ultimately make yoga more accessible to the male massive. It's about starting a new conversation about yoga, and to change the way guys see it today in the Western world.

The goal is simple: smash the stereotype and get more guys on the mat.

Even today, yoga is stigmatised. It is still seen as something for the girls – your sister, your girlfriend, your mum and their friends. It's easy to see on social media and in Western media that yoga is a feminine pastime. But did you know that yoga was originally just for men?

Regardless of the old ways or the new stereotypes the truth is, yoga is great for everybody and every body. Its benefits are undeniable, and it has no gender, colour, race, age or physical requirement.

Yoga gives you whatever you need. It can make you sweat and challenge your body; it can alleviate pain, tension or tightness; it can calm the mind, ease anxiety and change the way you see the world around you. Yoga isn't just a thing you do on the mat for an hour a day; it's a lifestyle, a philosophy and a way to connect to ourselves, to each other and the world we live in.

When I started BOYS OF YOGA, I never thought it would turn into a global movement of this

'YOGA IS GREAT FOR EVERYBODY AND EVERY BODY. THE BENEFITS ARE UNDENIABLE'

magnitude. It has been an amazing journey and one I'm continually inspired by every single day.

This book, like my teachings, is simply to share my own experiences in a way I believe to be true and to translate the wisdom of the practice I have learned over the years in a way that is easy to digest. I hope this speaks to you, just like the practice did to me when I started yoga. There is nothing in this book that says what is right and wrong. It is merely ideas, considerations and my experiences. All the photos and words are my own and all the stories belong to the BOYS that have joined me in helping to smash the stereotype of yoga that persists in the Western world. From pro-surfers to DJs, stay-at-home fathers to industry executives, graphic designers to plumbers, all the BOYS in this book, and so many more, come from all walks of life and from all around the world. Yoga doesn't have a type – it just is.

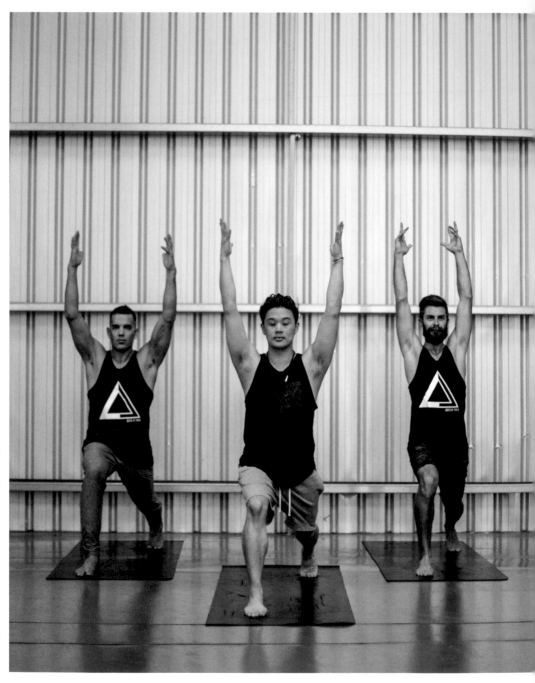

Left to right: Dustin Brown, Michael James Wong, Benny Gould

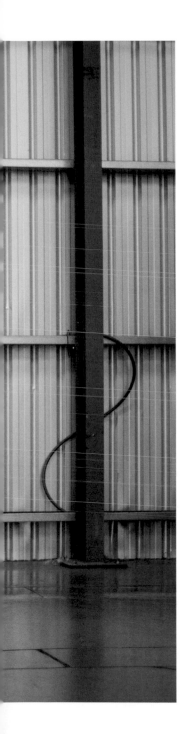

This is a book with purpose: to get more guys onto the mat through education and communicating the value of yoga. In these pages you'll find techniques about where to start and how to get going, and keep going.

We all know a guy who needs to start yoga. Or maybe you are that guy. The biggest issue we have with yoga today isn't the practice, but the word itself. For those just starting out, or those not quite ready to start, know that yoga will benefit your life, you just have to be ready and willing to give it a try. And if you've made it this far by picking up this book, you've already done the hardest part: you've started. Taking the first step is always the toughest part of doing anything new.

My biggest wish is that this book helps get you or your brother, boyfriend, dad, work colleague, sceptic or whoever onto the mat for the first time.

The yoga will do the rest.

'YOGA WILL BENEFIT YOUR LIFE, YOU JUST HAVE TO BE WILLING TO GIVE IT A TRY'

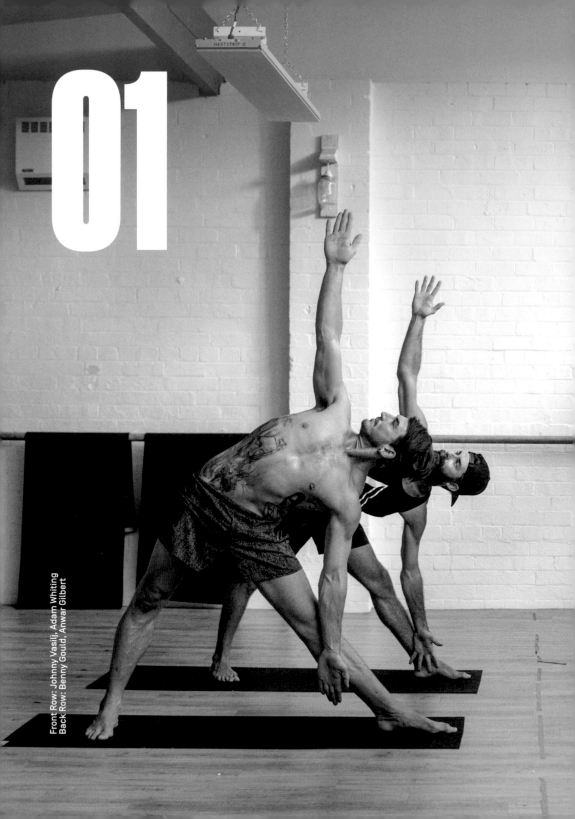

01

Front Row: Johnny Vasili, Adam Whiting
Back Row: Benny Gould, Anwar Gilbert

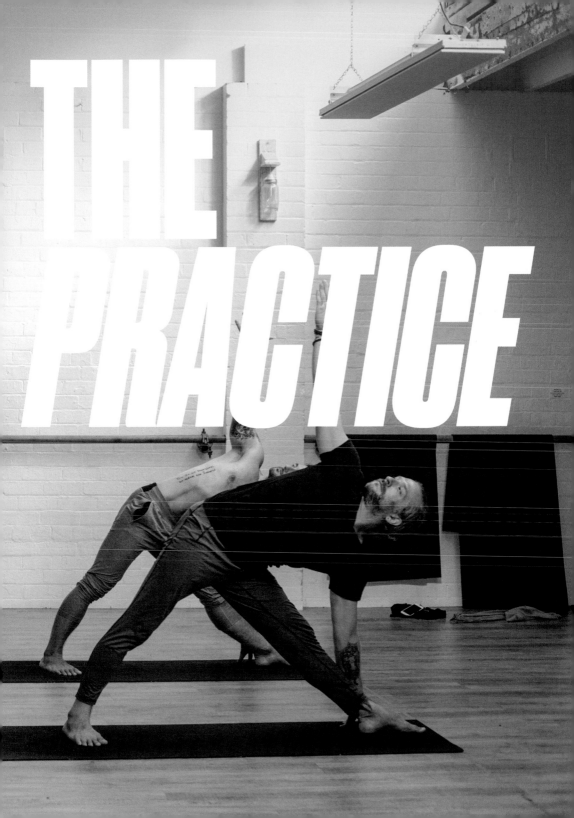

THE PRACTICE

What Is Yoga All About?

We live in a world that is always
on – online, on loud, on show,
on high alert. In today's society,
we're overloaded with things to
do, meetings to be had, calls to be
made and coffees to be shared.
We thrive on busy schedules, busy
lives and just the idea itself of being
busy. We talk more than listen. We
speed up without ever thinking
about slowing down. We've become
accustomed to thinking that this is
how life is meant to be.

But a growing number of us are starting to see that maybe it's time to turn the volume down and step into something less chaotic.

Over the past decade yoga has become increasingly popular in the Western world. These days it feels like there is a yoga studio popping up on every street corner and pretty soon there will be more of them than Starbucks branches in America alone (we can only hope). Look around and you'll see that yoga is now in the mainstream, helping lead the wellness revolution, and it's about time. The world is starting to wake up to the benefits of the practice and a more mindful way of living. But don't be fooled into thinking that yoga is some new fad. Yoga has been around for thousands of years, and it'll be around for thousands more to come. Right now, as yoga enjoys its place in the zeitgeist, it's a great time to pay attention and get started.

It's hard to miss the conversation because it is everywhere: yoga is mindful movement; it is functional mobility for our bodies; it is calming for our minds; it is everything we want and need it to be. This all might sound too good to be true, or come cloaked in language you find unfamiliar, but getting started is much easier than you might think.

You might not realise it, but you're probably already doing it.

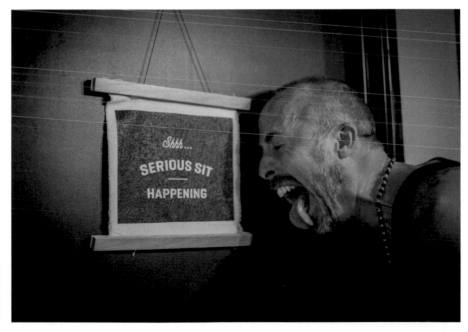

Scott Schwenk

So You Say I'm Already Doing Yoga?

As children, most of us spent our time playing, running around and getting dirty in the outdoors. We didn't take life too seriously. We acted the fool and liked to have a good time, no matter the consequences. It's also likely that when we got angry or frustrated our parents taught us to take a few deep breaths to calm down (usually after being sent to our rooms).

This is yoga. You just might have been calling it by a different name.

Think back to when you were younger. You played football, basketball, hockey, rugby or some other sport. You'd wake up on game day and head to the field ready to play. But when you got there, you didn't just run on the field and jump straight in. It's likely you started with a team talk, a moment when you aligned your focus and talked about intentions, such as trying your best and working together. You did a few stretches, nothing too vigorous; just a few minutes to warm up the entire body, become aware of the moment and move simply.

This is yoga. You just might have been calling it by a different name.

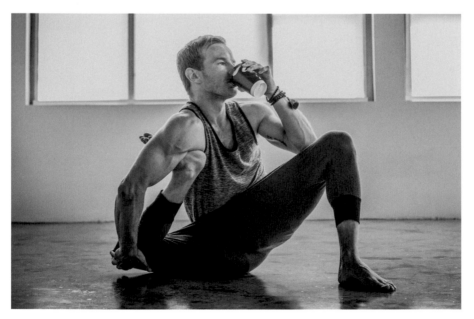

Davin Jones

'THIS IS YOGA. YOU JUST MIGHT HAVE BEEN CALLING IT BY A DIFFERENT NAME'

Or when you wake up at home, ready for the day ahead, you don't just pop up from the mattress and run out the door. It's likely you take a moment to stretch the arms, move the body gently, roll out the neck a few times and ease yourself into the day.

This is yoga. You just might have been calling it by a different name.

Try to remember a time recently when you've been angry or frustrated. It might be when someone cut you off on the road or you didn't get the job you wanted or your next-door neighbour decided to throw a party on a week night. You may have wanted to scream out a few choice words or throw your middle finger in the air in protest. But you stopped, took a breath, chose to be the bigger person and just let it go.

This is yoga. You just might have been calling it by a different name.

Physically, yoga is a dynamic stretching of the body. Off the mat, it's not taking life too seriously; it's slowing down, taking deep breaths, fighting frustration, keeping a level head, calming the mind, easing social tension, living in the moment, strengthening your focus, enhancing your relationships, learning to communicate, dealing with stress, overcoming challenges, living in the now, paying attention to what you're doing, caring deeply and taking the time to breathe.

If you can relate to any of the above, then you're already doing yoga. You just might have been calling it by a different name.

What Does Yoga Actually Mean?

Specifically, yoga means 'union'. It is translated from the classical Indian language of Sanskrit as 'yuj', or 'yoke', like that which is used to connect an ox to a cart. In Western translation, yoga is a connection: to our bodies, minds and breath; to each other and the world around us.

So to practise yoga is to connect, on all levels. If you're on the mat, connect with what you're doing and how you're breathing: every action and pose. Don't just 'do' the poses. Feel them. Notice the details – push, pull, ground and lift – feel the muscles engage, feel the floor, feel it all. Connect to every bit of the body in action. It's often said that yoga on the mat is meditation in motion.

If you're off the mat, connect with the conversation you're in, put your phone down and pay attention, be mindful in your actions, acknowledge your feelings and emotions, be nice to others, listen like you mean it, stop talking so much and treat everyone you meet with kindness.

This is yoga.

Travis Eliot, Los Angeles

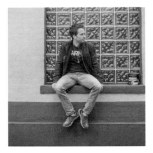

'Yoga is freedom. Every human being is looking for freedom. Some do it through negative means and others do it through positive means. But we all want to be free. And yoga helps us achieve this.'

Josh Blau, Melbourne

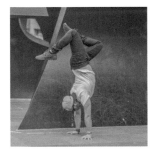

'Yoga is union. Pure bliss. Happiness. A way to be at peace with everything that is happening around you. Calm in the eye of the storm.'

Ude Okoye, London

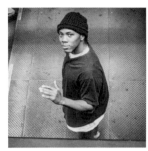

'Yoga is the thing that brings me to the present, into a place of appreciation for that moment. For me, it's a cure-all. If you haven't done it, you should try it.'

Victor Chau, Hong Kong

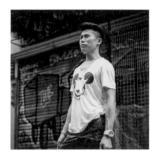

'Yoga is living, being 100 per cent aware.'

Kyle Gray, Glasgow

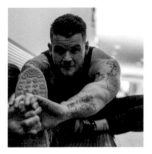

'Yoga is the practice of knowing yourself.'

Eric Ernerstedt, Sweden

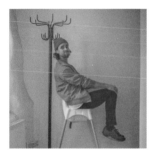

'Yoga is taking responsibility for your happiness.'

Octavio Salvado, Bali

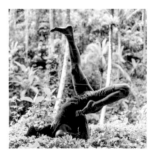

'Yoga is the greatest way to refine my authenticity and discover who I am. It is the ultimate battleground. It is not a place for the weak of heart; it's far too confrontational for that.'

Adam Husler, London

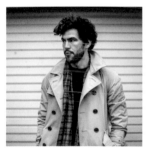

'Yoga is the practice of self-enquiry, through the control of movement and breath. It is an entirely subjective experience.'

MEET THE BOYS
JASE TE PATU
NEW ZEALAND

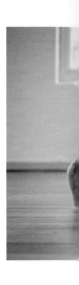

What's your story? I'm from humble beginnings. I was raised with my younger bro by my grandparents. My parents split when I was two years old. I only met my mum in 2014. Not knowing your real parents creates some pretty deep self-belief from a young age. I was raised in both the Māori and Anglo-Saxon ways, as my grandparents were native speakers and steeped in the traditional ways of our indigenous people. I was encouraged to try anything and everything. My 'A-type' personality meant I achieved quite a lot at a young age. I represented New Zealand in three sports and won a scholarship to school.

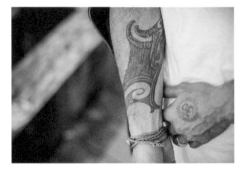

All of those achievements left me exhausted, though. I remember being at my 40th birthday and my friend said to me, 'What are you good at now?' I realised I had been DOING life rather than BEING it! Two years later and I'm enjoying life much more, having taken my foot off the pedal – more yin and less yang!

What do you most value in others? I admire 'presence' in a person. That to me is true connection, true yoga off the mat. Please put your iPhone/iPad/laptop down before you talk to me. I will give you my full attention if you give me yours.

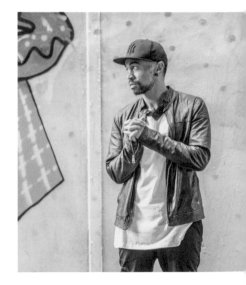

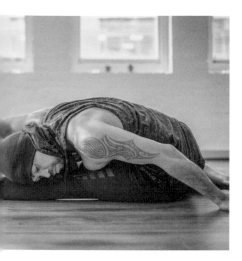

What would make you skip practice? If the All Blacks are playing, I'm out. I'm in front of my mate's big screen, losing my voice, yelling the house down – shameless!

What advice would you give to someone stepping onto the mat for the first time? Breathe and drop the judgement. We land on our mat with so many expectations – of ourselves, of the teacher. Once we drop the judgement, we are able to be completely in the body and breath.

Which pose do you really hate? Gomukhasana (Cow Face pose). Trying to wrap these big Māori Rugby legs into that posture is not ideal.

People think that, as a guy, I'll be less interested in the traditional philosophies and prefer doing handstands. When I speak about the *Gita* or *Patanjali's Sutras* or teach a Yin class, people lean in to listen to what I have to say. There's more to this guy than my tattoos, muscles, handstands and splits.

WORDSMITH.
WARRIOR.
P.L.A.Y.ER.
YOGI.

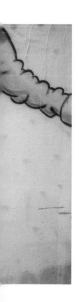

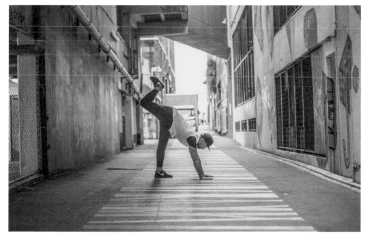

@warriorjase
Read more at boysofyoga.com @boysofyoga

MEET THE BOYS

LES LEVENTHAL

CALIFORNIA

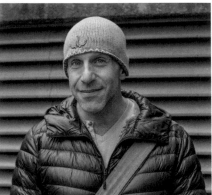

What's your story? I'm officially a gypsy nomad – I'm American and I taught in San Francisco for a decade and then Bali for over three years, and now I'm teaching all over this amazing world, from Australia to Europe to the Middle East – places that have small communities and need the yoga as well as those crazy, large festivals.

What did you want to be growing up? A gold-medal-winning Olympic swimmer because I was good at it and I was raised to believe that winning equals happiness.

What do you value most in others? The truth – it doesn't waste anyone's time.

What does a male yogi look like? Like every man that walks this earth. Guys don't do yoga because they think it's light and fairy. Not with me. We're gonna dig deeper. That's what we come for, to journey to those places.

PAIN IN THE ASS. CHURRO EATER. SPORTS JUNKIE. YOGI.

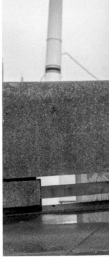

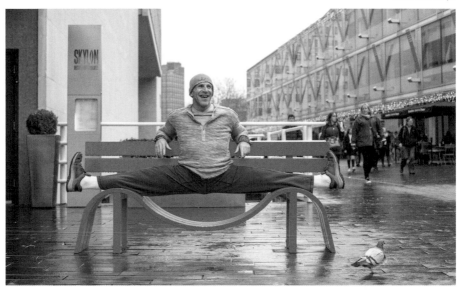

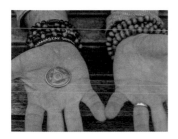

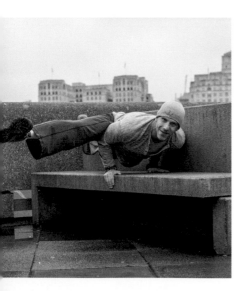

What are the biggest stereotypes about guys who do yoga? That they're only good if the man bun looks just right. Yoga relaxes all those external expectations about what I should look like or sound like as a man doing yoga.

What was the biggest challenge when you started the practice? I was smoking again. I didn't like who I was. I was back out drinking and using when I found yoga. My negative body image and self-consciousness were raging. So, my biggest challenge was just to stay alive and not do further harm to myself. I've had some brushes with suicide and this was not a happy time in my life, and the gift and the challenge was that there was no one for me to lay blame on.

There is hope. Transformation is possible. But I can't just pray for God to do that for me. I have to put in the work.

@lesleventhalyoga
Read more at boysofyoga.com @boysofyoga

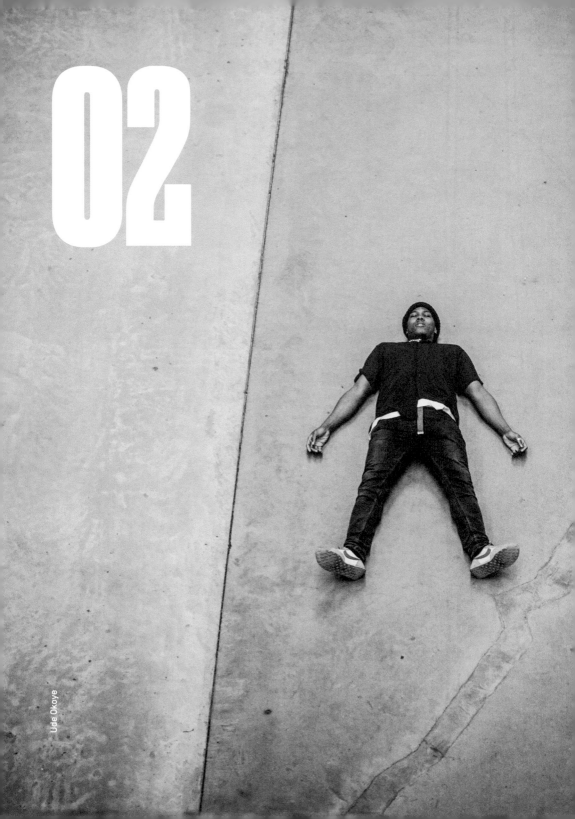

02

Ude Okoye

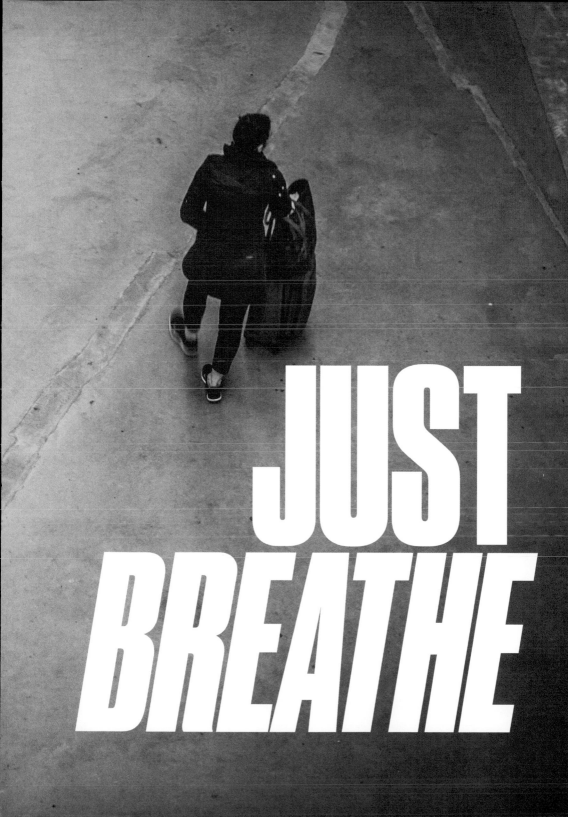

**You're One Breath
Away From Calm**

Did you know that the average
person takes between 12 and
20 breaths a minute? Over the
course of a day, that's 17,000–
30,000 breaths. That's a lot.
   We breathe when we sleep
and when we eat. We breathe
when we're on the bus and
we breathe more when we're
chasing it. As long as we are
alive we are always breathing.
But how often are we really
thinking about it?

How often are we giving our breath the attention it deserves?

Breathing is automatic. It just happens. Sure, it's keeping you alive, but that's no big deal, right?

The amazing thing about breathing is that when you choose to focus on it and take the time to notice it, you get so much more out of it. So maybe it's time to start paying more attention to the breath.

We can all relate to times in our lives when things have gotten a bit messy or out of control, and these are the times when the breath is our biggest asset. One deep breath can help alleviate a whole world of chaos.

When I was 18, I was living in Los Angeles and I had asked my friend Brandon to teach me how to drive a manual car. Driving manual wasn't a common thing in LA when I was growing up, so I wanted to learn. From the moment I got in, it felt like there was way too much going on: three pedals for my feet; one hand on the steering wheel and the other hand on the gear stick. I had to look with my eyes, listen with my ears and deal with about a hundred and one other things going on around me on the road. It was complete chaos.

But in one of those first lessons, Brandon simply said, 'If you put your foot on the brake, no matter what else is happening, the car will slow down and everything will be ok. Then you can decide what's best from there.' Fifteen years later and I've never forgotten this.

And that's how the breath works. No matter the chaos that's around you, just remember that if you stop and take a deep breath, everything will slow down. Then you can decide what's best from there.

'ONE DEEP BREATH CAN HELP ALLEVIATE A WHOLE WORLD OF CHAOS'

The Breath Is Life. Respect It

When used with the right approach, the breath has the power to calm our minds, ease our anxiety and appease our anger. The breath is transformational, and the best thing about it is that it's always there (and it's free!).

The breath gives us the support to do the things we want to do in our lives and it will never let you down if you give it the respect it deserves.

I've been lucky (or unlucky) enough to know the value of the breath since I was very young. I'm asthmatic and I carry around a little blue inhaler that helps relieve my airways when I have an attack. I've had trouble breathing since I was very young, and there are times, even today, when I literally can't get the breath in; a simple inhale and exhale feels like I'm sucking a peanut through a bendy straw. Unless you also suffer with asthma, you'll never know

the fear that comes with simply trying to breathe.

For me, breathing is not something to take lightly. (The sad part here for all the asthmatics reading this is that there isn't a magic moment coming up where I say, 'And yoga will cure your asthma!') However, over the years yoga has gone a long way to helping me control my anxiety around it. The breath is a tool that can physically calm, emotionally ease and spiritually invigorate. You just have to know how to use it.

Remember that breathing is simple: it's an inhale and an exhale. Approaching each and every breath one at a time reminds us to live in the now. Yogis will say that life only exists within the space of the inhale and exhale, and to ignore this is to ignore true living. So the longer the breath, the more we are putting into living.

Most of us forget to value the breath. It becomes an afterthought and often we don't honour its purpose. A lack of integrity in the body, much like the breath, will only lessen its benefit to your life and the things you want to do. Don't wait until it's compromised to prioritise it.

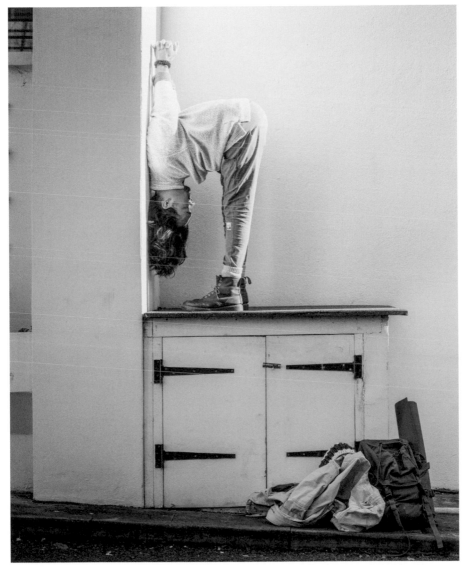

Jake Paul White

Omar Sultani

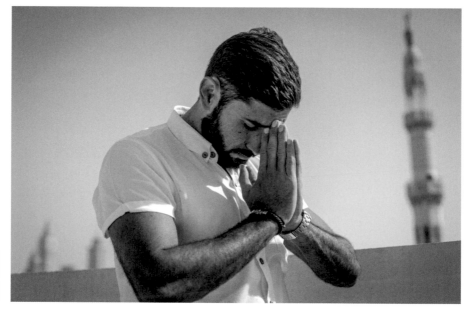

Go Deep, Go Slow

'Take a few deep breaths ...'

I bet you've heard this phrase once or twice before in your life. Maybe your other half said it to you after someone royally screwed you over. Maybe your colleagues have said it after your manager yelled at you unnecessarily.

Taking a deep breath has immense value. It can be like a warm and comforting hug you didn't know you needed. It's the support you want, the space you need and the permission to know that everything is going to be ok (and the world will not end).

In yoga the breath is everything: it's the first thing we do and the last thing we let go. We lead with the breath in the first pose, the last pose and every pose in between.

How To Take A Deep Breath

Do you actually know how to take a deep breath?

It's funny how we all have a tendency to say, 'Of course I do.'

But to be honest, I didn't until I was taught. The truth was that I'd never really thought that hard about it.

Do I open my mouth or keep it closed?

Do I fill up my belly or my chest?

How slow is 'slow' for the inhale and for the exhale?

These are all questions many of us ask when we really think about it.

For me, I believe slow is the way to go. Slowing down the breath gives you time to appreciate the inhale and exhale, the quality of breath and its value to every moment of your day. In yoga, like life, first we breathe, then we do everything else.

Regardless which technique you choose to use, every breath you take has four parts.

The first two are easy.

Part 1: The inhale. The air enters the body through the nose.

Part 2: The exhale. The air exits the body through the nose.

The last two are a little more subtle.

Part 3: The space at the top of the inhale where no more breath enters.

Part 4: The space at the bottom of the exhale where no more breath exits.

The spaces at the top and bottom of the breath are where we find the calm. They're our escape from the chaos. It's in these gaps that we're not distracted by what's coming and going and we're in the now. They are the still point. This is how we find quiet, and the breath is the gateway into the silence.

Take a moment and give it a try.

Inhale, pause, exhale, pause, repeat. It was a real mind-blowing, life-changing moment for me when I first learned this. If you're lucky enough to have learned this already, then keep doing what you're doing and just breathe.

The Breathing Techniques

There are a few breathing (pranayama) techniques that will help you on and off the yoga mat, and in this book we'll talk about three specifically. While there are many techniques, each with their own purpose and value, it's good to learn a few basics that will serve you well in everyday life.

When practising these techniques for the first time, find yourself a comfortable position, cross-legged on the floor, or sitting easily in a chair. Don't overcomplicate it and just focus on the inhale and exhale, no matter the technique.

These are just a few of many breathing techniques. If you find they are helpful and valuable, then continue to do them as often as you can.

Go slow, be gentle and don't overthink it.

Just breathe.

The Box Breath

This technique is focused on balance and support. It's simple and not forced. Breathe in long, slow and deep; breathe out long, slow and deep.

How to do it

- Inhale to the count of four, mouth closed, evenly drawing the breath in through the nose, letting the air wash across the back of the throat, filling the chest and lungs from the front to back (not bottom to top). Imagine blowing up a balloon, rather than filling up a glass of water. This will minimise unneeded movement in the body.

- Pause effortlessly and hold for the count of four.

- Exhale to the count of four, mouth closed, evenly moving the breath out and warming the back of the lips as it exits the nose.

- Pause effortlessly and hold for the count of four.

- Repeat with ease until you feel calm.

The Victorious Breath

Referred to in yoga as the Ujjayi breath, this technique focuses on energising the body, filling you up with an empowering and vibrant life force. This is one of the most commonly taught breathing techniques in a yoga class and is a great tool for courage, motivation and creating some internal heat as you practise.

This breath is strong, warming and uplifting.

How to do it

- Inhale with the mouth closed, deeply and vigorously drawing the breath in through the nose and across the back of the throat, filling up the chest and lungs from the front to back (see the Box Breath).

- When you're ready to exhale, empty the lungs, with the mouth closed, warming and heating the breath as it escapes, the same way you would fog up a mirror. Retain a slight constriction in the back of the throat.

- Continue and repeat.

The Lion's Breath

This technique is about letting go – the euphoria of the release. This is an open-mouthed, let-it-all-go type of breath. And it feels pretty damn good. Most people have a tendency to hold on to too much inside – we keep things bottled up and never let them go.

This breath reminds us that, often, it's better out than in.

How to do it

- Inhale with the mouth closed, deeply and vigorously drawing the breath in through the nose and across the back of the throat, filling up the chest and lungs front to back (see the Box Breath).

- Pause, don't hold the breath but prepare to release.

- To exhale, open the mouth, stick out the tongue and push the breath out in one strong release.

- Pause and repeat until you feel calmer, lighter and refreshed. You can't overdose on this technique.

Just Breathe

Now that you have these three techniques, try them out and see which works well for you. You will find that at different times, a different technique serves best. Remember, you take between 12 and 20 breaths in a minute, so you've got a lot of opportunities to try them out.

There is one certainty in life: if you don't breathe, you will die. To live to the fullest is to breathe to the fullest.

So when things go right or things go wrong, just breathe.

When you're not feeling your best, just breathe.

When things are fast and need to slow down, just breathe.

At the end of the day, no matter the situation, just breathe.

Sjaak Van Tunen

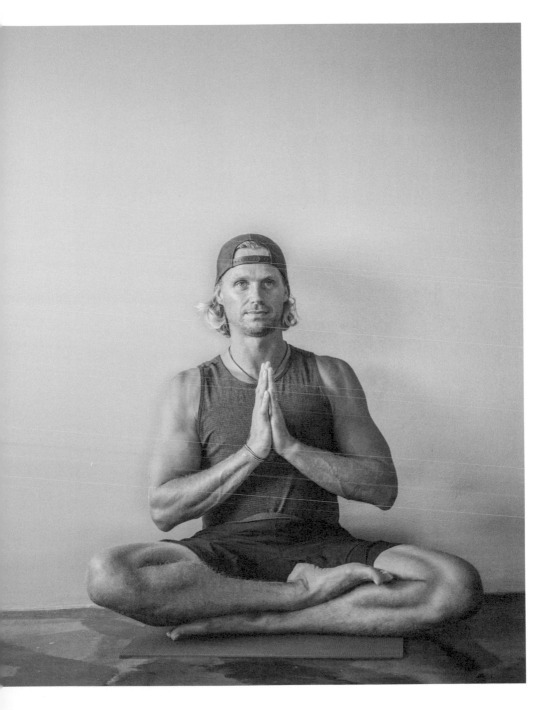

MEET THE BOYS

YANCY SCOT SCHWARTZ

NEW YORK

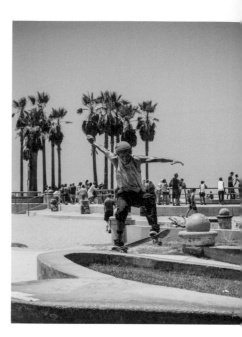

What's your story? I was born in Queens, New York. My dad was from Brooklyn, my mum was from Ecuador. My mum was a babysitter and my dad a maintenance man – he was a masterful electrician. We had our apartment for free so my parents were able to save some money. They rented out the spare room, so growing up I had a lot of kids and strangers in and out of the apartment. My dad was very mellow, super quiet. My mum was very strict and her discipline could be very physical. At a young age I became interested in skateboarding and that ruled my life. It was eat, sleep, skate back then.

We've all got a few stories that we aren't the most proud of. Care to share one? When I was 17 I ran away from home. My mum had gone back to South America so I ran away to California with a drug-addicted girl and stayed there for a year or so. I told my dad I would be gone for a week but I didn't come back for over a year.

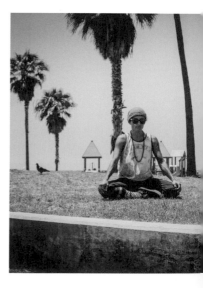

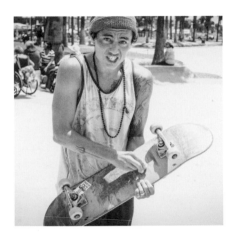

What's the best and worst relationship you've ever had? Skateboarding. It's gratifying and it's an elite community, but it's an unforgiving art. I've broken bones and had surgery. It's a risky way of life.

What was the biggest challenge when you first started practising yoga? My ego. Letting it go in order to do the class was very challenging. I had to learn to let that part go and keep practising, with no expectations.

People expect you to be strong all the time – both emotionally and physically. Sometimes I want to throw my hands up in the air and give up.

But I must go on.

What's your favourite quote? 'When you can control your mouth, what goes into it, what comes out of it, then you have already mastered much of your mind.' Sri Dharma Mittra

PRO-SKATER.
VEGAN.
DHARMA JUNKIE.
YOGI.

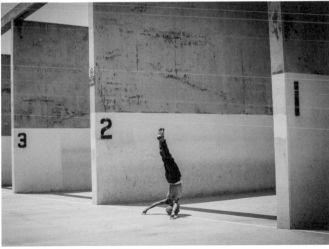

@yancyscotschwartz
Read more at boysofyoga.com @boysofyoga

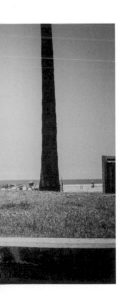

MEET THE BOYS

CHRIS MAGEE

IRELAND

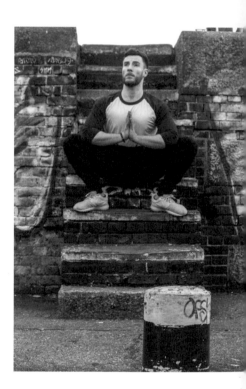

What's your story? I was born and raised in Northern Ireland. As a kid, I was always very active and creative, practising martial arts and playing team sports from around six or seven. I enjoyed learning, so I liked school and got along pretty well in everything I tried.

In my teens I continued to be heavily involved in sports, primarily rugby, and with that came a lot of weight training. By the time I was 18 I had a long list of injuries. My body was battered! Trapped nerves, muscle tears, dislocations – you name it, I probably had it.

How would your mother describe you? I asked her and she said 'handsome, hard-working and ambitious: a go-getter'. But, sure, mothers are always biased.

What do you most value in others and why?
Honesty. We live in a world of false appearances – social-media personas and artificial communications. To meet someone and interact openly and honestly is a rare and wonderful thing.

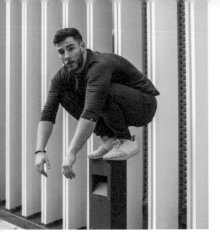

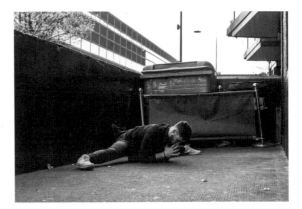

GUINNESS MAN.
ACTOR.
EX-STEAK-LOVER.
YOGI.

We've all done a few things we aren't too proud of. Care to share one? One night, when I was younger, I got really drunk and peed on the door of a police station ... not my brightest moment!

Why do you keep coming back to the mat? It has become much more of a mental practice for me: time to clear the mind and bring focus and awareness to myself that I can then take into life off the mat.

Tell us about a time your yoga practice came into play off the mat? I was a bit of a hothead when I was younger and got into a few scrapes. As time progressed, that anger manifested itself in other forms, like road rage. It was always seemingly small stuff that set me off big time. My yoga practice comes into play off the mat every day when a scenario like this arises and I can let that stuff go.

What is your personal mantra? Life is all about balance.

@mageesy
Read more at boysofyoga.com @boysofyoga

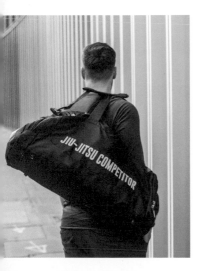

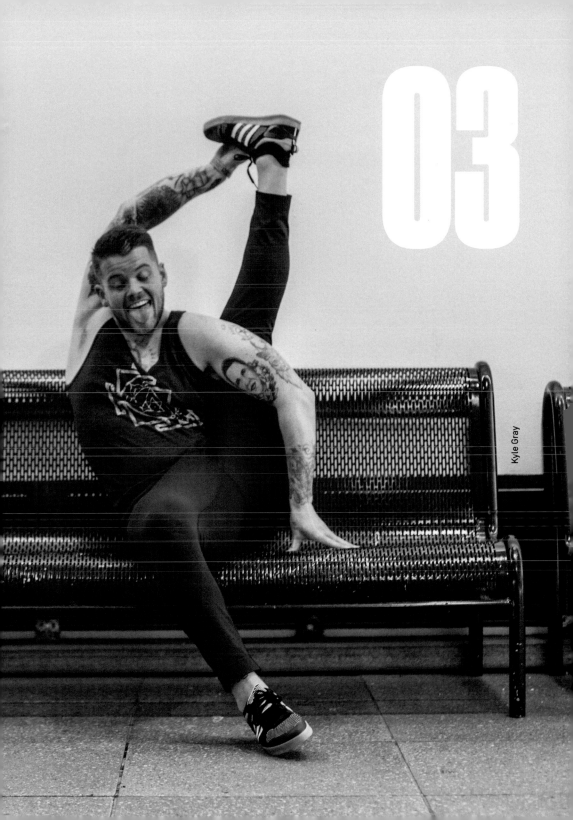

03

Kyle Gray

Learning The Basics
And How To Get Started

The first time you go to a yoga class
it can feel quite daunting. It seems
like a whole a new language, with all
kinds of funny words and instructions
that ask you to put your arms and
legs in places they've never been
before. If you're anything like me
when I started, you're sweating from
places you didn't know could, using
muscles you didn't know you had
and, to top it off, the teacher is telling
you to calm down and control your
breath when all you can think is, we
need more oxygen in this room!

While these days everyone tells you you should go to a class, no one actually tells you how to get started, as in 'blank sheet of paper, what exactly goes where?' getting started.

This is the chapter where we'll look at answering some of the practical questions for anyone brand new to yoga. Simply put: what goes where, so I know what I'm doing?

For yogis who practise regularly, we often forget those first few times on the mat. But it's important to remember that everyone was a beginner at one point. Every single guy in this book, every single yogi in class, every single person who seems like they've got it figured out – they too were in your shoes once. They were a beginner just like you. And what they all did, just like you're going to do, is take those shoes off, get on the mat and try.

The best advice I was given when I started yoga was: 'Don't worry. No one is looking at you. Everyone is too busy worrying about themselves to care about you.' I'm thankful for that advice; it got me through a lot of those early classes.

Another point I want to mention is that yoga, or the 'asana', which is the physical part of yoga (making shapes with the body – left foot here, right foot there), will look different in every person's body, and there is no one definitive way to do any pose. There is no right or wrong way to do the postures.

The poses will look different, but more importantly feel different, every day. Take a moment to think about your week so far: what you've done and what you haven't. Have you run five miles today? Have you sat at your desk for the last 12 hours or have you been horizontal on the sofa, binge-watching your favourite Netflix series? No two days are the same, and every day your body will feel different because you've done different things. And so your yoga practice will look and feel different too. Never judge today against yesterday. All that matters is today. Drop everything else.

The beauty of yoga is that it will teach you that there is no perfect pose or ideal outcome. It's not how it looks; it's how it feels.

It's all yoga, however it comes out.

Stop Making Excuses

'I can't go to yoga. I'm not flexible enough.'

This is one of the many excuses I hear from guys all the time. If you stop and think about it, it's absurd. It's like saying, 'I can't go to the kitchen, I'm too hungry' or, 'I can't take a shower, I'm just too dirty'. Yoga is the remedy for aches and pains and lack of mobility in the body. Once you start your physical practice, the body will get stronger, the muscles more malleable, the hips more flexible. Tying your own shoelaces will be something you'll be able to do well into your old age.

Truth be told, the biggest issue isn't even the practice. It's walking through the door that first time, fighting the fear or embarrassment and just getting on with it. For so many guys, fear of expectation stops us from even trying. Remember, you're doing something new and different. It's not going to go exactly to plan, and that's the best part. We get caught in our head, thinking we need to be 'good' and perform a certain way in class. Don't let the fear of 'not being good' or 'not doing it right' stop you from even starting. There is no such thing as being good at yoga. It's not a thing.

Sadly, the guys coming up with excuses for why they can't start are the ones who will miss out most. It's the ego making decisions that aren't in their best interest.

Yoga isn't about touching your toes; it's about what you learn on the way down.

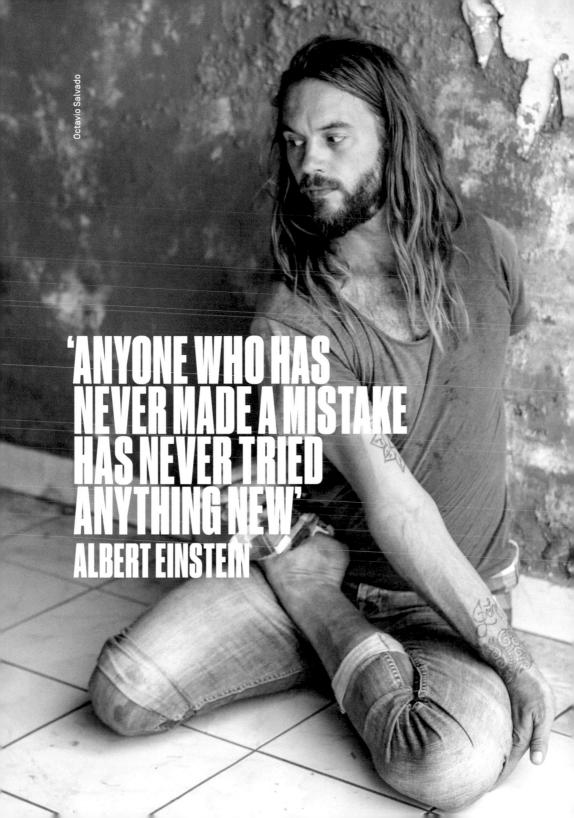

'ANYONE WHO HAS NEVER MADE A MISTAKE HAS NEVER TRIED ANYTHING NEW'

ALBERT EINSTEIN

Octavio Salvado

Let's Get Started

When you're ready to go to class – or if you're just looking for a few tips and techniques – know that there are some yoga basics that will really help you get started. Before you walk into the studio it's important to know what you're working with. Some guys are tall and thin, while others are short and stocky, with plenty more somewhere in the middle. If you cycle or run, you may have really tight hip flexors and hamstrings; if you lift heavy weights at the gym, you may have tight shoulders and low range of motion in your chest and upper spine. These aren't bad things – they're just *your* things, and it's important to be aware of them when you start your yoga practice.

A house is built on strong foundations, and so should your yoga practice be
There are three key things that make up the foundations of your practice: the breath, the body and the intention. Each has a purpose that will help you as you start doing more yoga.

'YOGA ISN'T ABOUT TOUCHING YOUR TOES; IT'S ABOUT WHAT YOU LEARN ON THE WAY DOWN'

The breath is always the priority. It's the fuel and the calm, a moment-by-moment reminder not to try so hard. *Breathe and then move.* If you remember this one simple phrase in yoga, you'll find that everything will get easier.

The body is your vehicle for the physical practice. There are a lot of moving parts. Move slow, feel everything and remember that the body is connected and all the parts must work together to get where you want to go.

The intention is the final component. It is the 'why' in your practice; we call it 'sankalpa'. Having an intention allows you to have purpose in your actions and a reason for being on the mat. It doesn't have to be a life-changing thing – even simple intentions will give your practice a sense of purpose.

Remember that yoga is a practice and there is process to the progress. Sometimes the more you want it, the harder it gets.

To learn, try, fly and fail at yoga poses is just a matter of experience. Physically, it builds strength and stamina, encourages us to breathe and manage our movements on the mat. Mentally and emotionally, it helps us to fight the fear and limitations that we put on ourselves, the ones that say 'we can't' or 'we're not good enough' or 'someone like us shouldn't do this'.

Here are a few intentions I like to use:

1. **I practise to quiet the busyness in my head.**

2. **I practise so I can tie my shoelaces when I'm older.**

3. **I practise to slow down, think less and feel more.**

When our intentions are strong, the pose becomes easier because we're approaching it for the right reasons.

What Stuff Do I Need For Class?

What do I wear, what do I bring?

It's easy to laugh about this, but it's a real concern when you're starting out. People don't tell you what to wear for class; they just assume you know.

The first time I went to a yoga class I wore board shorts and a baggy cotton shirt. Bad move. Board shorts are only good for catching sweat and water, but get them too wet and it'll feel like you're cutting off your circulation to your upper thighs – and other regions. At that point you'd be better off in your underwear, but that's probably not the best look or the most appropriate.

After that first mishap, I thought, *Hey, I'll wear sweatpants*. Again, another bad move. Despite their name, sweatpants aren't actually that great for sweating in. Awkward and cumbersome would be a good way of describing the experience. The next time I went to class, I thought, *Pyjama pants!* They were lightweight and comfortable,

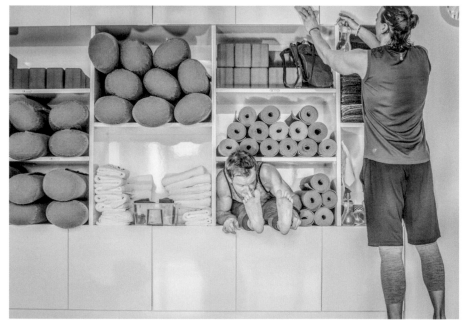

Davin Jones (left), Cristian Blanch

easy to move in and you could feel the breeze through them. But when I got to the studio that day, I thought, *I'm in my pyjama pants, in public, going to a yoga class, not having a clue what I'm doing.* You might as well have just grabbed a big foam finger and stood next to me with a sign that said 'I'm with stupid'. Yeah, it felt like that.

These days, there are lots of good options available to you. You can actually buy yoga clothes specifically for guys, but these aren't absolutely necessary, and you can wait until it makes sense before you invest.

For me, I've found that some of the best things to wear are what we already have at home, and top of the list are football or running shorts and a form-fitted cotton T-shirt or tank top.

Football or running shorts are great when you're starting because lots of guys have a pair at home, even if they don't get worn that often, and, if not, they can be bought pretty cheaply from a sports store. They are short enough so that they don't drag over the knees, and lightweight enough to give you the freedom to move. They're also usually made from material that doesn't hold onto the sweat.

Ideally, you don't want anything baggy on your top half because it will get in the way. There are a lot of poses like forward bends and downward-facing dog where a big, baggy T-shirt will suffocate you. Some guys go shirtless; this is ok and allowed in most classes, though do ask your teacher first. Do what works for you. You want your clothes to provide minimal distraction.

Ditch the socks
You don't need them. You may think you do, assuming they will help you grip the mat better, but the truth is they'll only get in the way. Going barefoot will ensure you don't slip and, more importantly, allow you to feel the connection to the floor, an essential part of the practice. Make it easy for yourself – leave the socks outside with your shoes. Less is more.

What about the mat?
In the old days yoga was done on animal skins, grass or dirt patches and, eventually, cotton blankets, rugs and carpet underlays. It wasn't until recently that the rubber mat was introduced – and we're very glad it's here now. A good, grippy mat will give you a huge amount of support. It will help you stay connected and steady and give you one

less distraction as you start to learn what goes where.

Most studios will have mats that you can borrow, so don't invest until you're ready, but know that there are many different types of mat that you can choose from. They are not 'one size fits all'.

If yoga becomes a regular thing, it's worth having your own mat. This way you become familiar with the surface and support it gives your practice. Another consideration is if other people sweat onto their mat as much as I do, I don't particularly want to spend an hour rolling around in it.

Sweaty support

People get sweaty. It's just a fact. When I first started I was embarrassed, I couldn't believe how much was pouring out of me. And in yoga it can be a distraction – it gets in your eyes and makes your arms and legs feel slippery. My best advice is to bring a towel and use it often. And remember, sweat is a natural way for the body to cleanse itself and rinse you out.

Give yourself props

Props are there to help. Using them doesn't mean you're worse than anyone else in the room; they're there to make the practice easier, and that's what it's all about. There are a multitude of different props you can choose from such as blocks, straps, bolsters and blankets. Choose wisely.

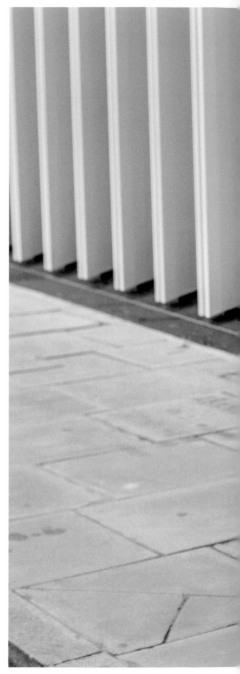

Chris Magee

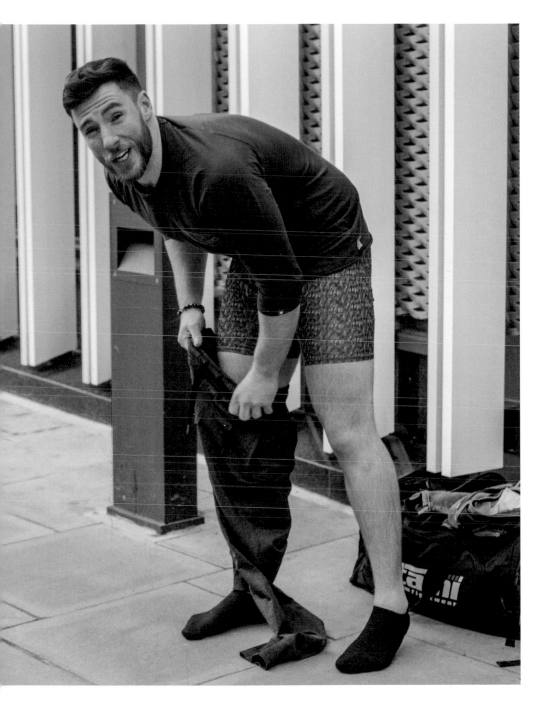

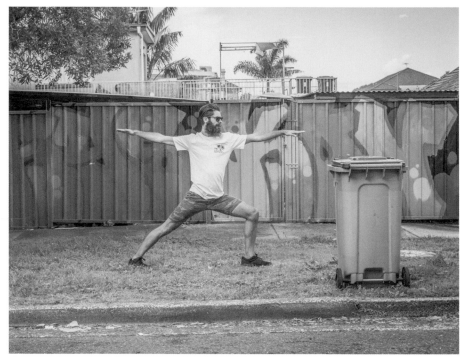

Benny Gould

The Poses You Need To Know

Like it or not, most public studio classes don't really cater to beginners. I mean real beginners (hold on, hear me out), like the ones who don't know the difference between a Downward-facing Dog and a Wiggly Panda (the latter isn't even a real pose). Studio classes can be tough for guys who are just trying

to keep up, but this doesn't mean you shouldn't go.

We've all been there, and so on the opposite page are a few good tips for newbies.

There are hundreds of poses in yoga, but learning some of the basic ones is a great place to start. Each of these poses is broken down into five points of focus, giving you the need-to-know information for what goes where and the key cues you need to get into the pose safely. (We've even added in the Sanskrit and phonetics to help you sound it out.)

Beginner's Checklist

1

Stay calm and take it slow

2

What goes where is more important than what it's called

3

Listen with your ears; look with your eyes

4

Don't do the pose; feel the pose

5

Don't compete; it's not about winning

6

Know that no one in the room is doing it 'perfectly'. They're just doing it differently

7

Do one thing at a time, not everything all at once

8

Don't forget to keep breathing

EASY POSE

Sukhasana *[soo-KAHS-anna]*

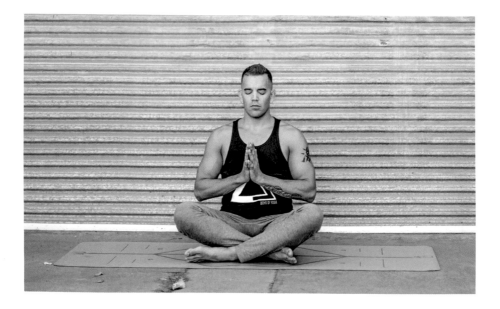

Easy pose is a common posture for meditation because the body is aligned, but at ease.

Five points of focus

1. Start seated, cross-legged, in a comfortable and grounded position.
2. Allow the sit bones to rest evenly as you sit tall through the spine.
3. Allow the shoulders to draw down the back, creating space around the neck.
4. Feel the back of the neck lengthen, the head stays level.
5. Place the hands together at the chest or comfortably on your lap.

CHILD'S POSE

Balasana *(bah-LAHS-anna)*

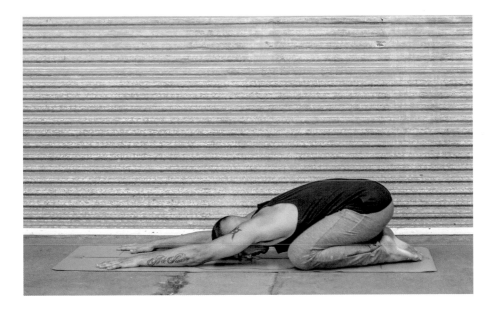

Child's pose is often the first pose of a class, allowing the body to soften and create stillness in the mind.

Five points of focus

1. Start face-down with knees wide and big toes touching.
2. Allow the hips to soften back towards the heels.
3. Rest the forehead towards the mat, but don't compress the neck.
4. Extend the hands forward to create length in the body, but draw the shoulders down the back to create space around the ears.
5. Close your eyes and relax into the pose.

COW POSE

Bitilasana *[bee-tee-LAHS-anna]*

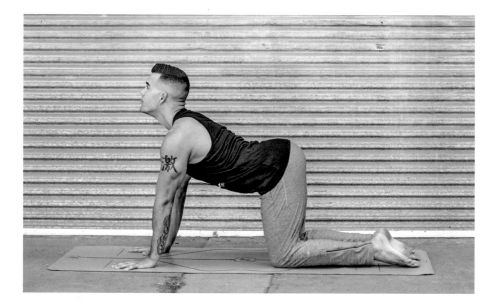

People often mix up Cat and Cow pose because the way they're instructed is opposite to the way they're practised; it should really be Cow and Cat pose! If in doubt, act like a scared cat or a mooing cow.

Five points of focus

1. From a table-top position, draw the chest forward and upward, broadening the collarbones as the shoulders draw down the back.
2. Ground the hands into the mat to create the necessary support.
3. Keep the neck in line with the spine.
4. Engage the core, drawing navel to spine, to support lower-back flexion.
5. Rotate the sit bones to the sky at the same time as the chest movement to move the lower spine.

CAT POSE

Marjaryasana *(marh-jahr-ee-AHS-anna)*

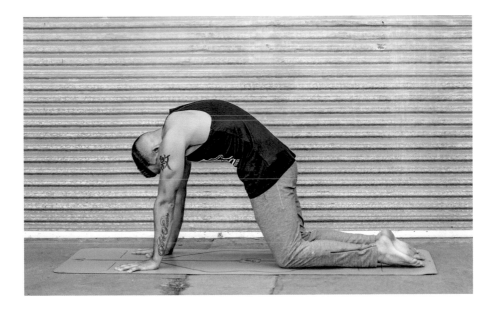

Cat and Cow poses should be done together as they are complementary, with the focus on gentle spinal flexion and extension.

Five points of focus

1. From a table-top position, press the hands into the mat, while arching the upper and middle spine.
2. Tuck the chin into the chest to elongate the back and neck.
3. Engage the core, drawing navel to spine, to support the back extension.
4. Lengthen the tailbone by spiralling the pelvis forward and down.
5. Move through multiple cycles of Cat and Cow together to warm and integrate the spine.

MOUNTAIN POSE

Tadasana *[tah-DAHS-anna]*

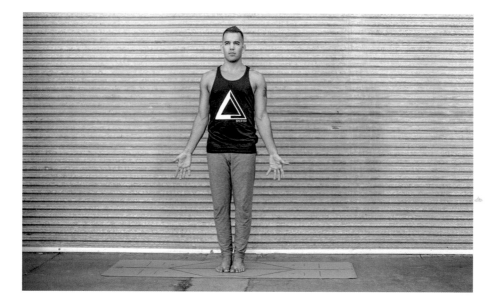

Mountain pose is the foundation for many poses. You can find elements of this pose in all asanas.

Five points of focus

1. Start standing with the feet together or slightly apart, placing even pressure into the mat.
2. Feel the shin bones draw into the midline of the body and the thighs internally rotate towards the back.
3. Keep a level pelvis and a tall spine.
4. Make space by drawing the shoulder blades down, leaving space for the neck to draw tall.
5. Extend the crown of your head to the sky and the fingertips towards the earth.

FORWARD FOLD

Uttanasana *[OOT-tan-AHS-anna]*

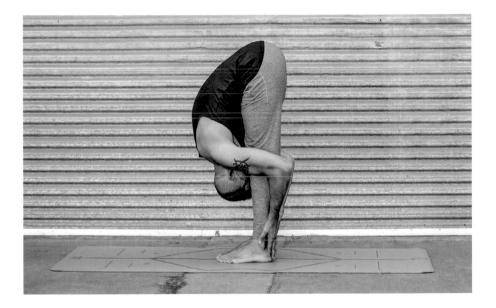

A simple forward fold is one of the most comprehensive stretches you can do to activate and engage the entire back line of the body.

Five points of focus

1. Fold the torso forward from the waist, allowing the spine to extend towards the mat.
2. Keep even pressure through the feet to support the body.
3. Keep a slight bend in the knees and tilt the sit bones towards the sky to lengthen the hamstrings.
4. Draw the shoulders down the back to make space around the ears.
5. Let the neck and head hang easily.

HALF FORWARD FOLD

Ardha Uttanasana *[ARE-dah OOT-tan-AHS-anna]*

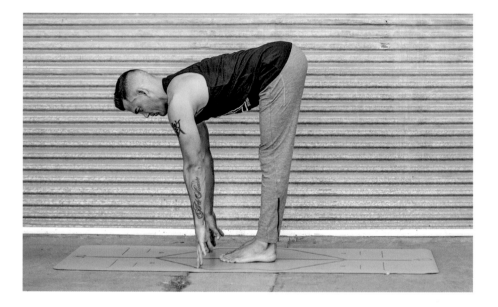

This pose helps to release the spine from a forward fold and activate, ready for movement.

Five points of focus

1. From a forward bend, bend the knees and lift the chest until it's parallel with the floor.
2. Broaden the collarbones as you draw the shoulders down the back.
3. Lengthen and elongate the spine.
4. Fix your gaze on the top edge of the mat, keeping the spine long.
5. Draw navel to spine, supporting the lower back.

FOUR-LIMBED STAFF POSE

Chaturanga Dandasana
[chaht-tour-ANG-ah dan-DAHS-anna]

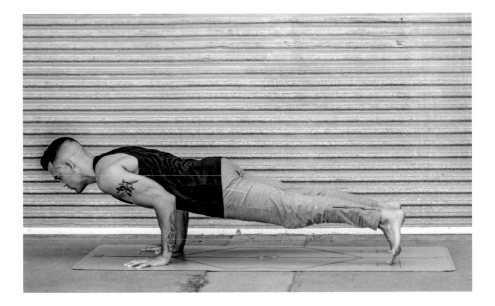

To modify this pose for an easier version, place your knees on the mat as you lower yourself down.

Five points of focus

1. Starting from a high plank position, create a steady base, stacking the shoulders above the wrist joints and with the hips slightly higher to keep the core active and legs engaged.
2. To transition, externally rotate the biceps forward as you move your chest forward and down, creating a 90-degree bend in the elbows.
3. The body stays in one line and moves together as one.
4. When lowered into the full pose, the shoulders and elbows should form a horizontal line, with the elbow and wrist of each arm in a vertical line.
5. The action of high to low plank is a smooth and fluid movement.

UPWARD-FACING DOG

Urdhva Mukha Svanasana
[oord-vah MOO-kah shvon-AHS-anna]

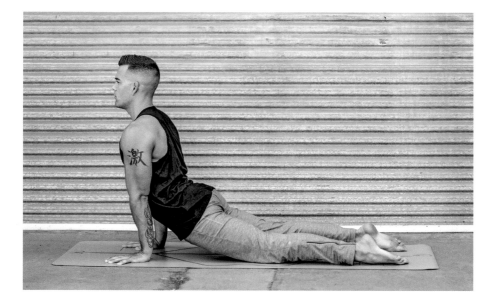

When doing this pose, think more about the heart opening than the back bending.

Five points of focus

1. Pressing through the tops of the feet, keep the knees and thighs lifted to protect the lower spine.
2. Pressing through the hands, draw the shoulders up, back and down, creating space in the front of the body.
3. Pull through the heels of the hands to open the heart space.
4. Keep the head and neck in line with the spine.
5. Engage the core by drawing navel to spine, for support.

DOWNWARD-FACING DOG

Adho Mukha Svanasana
[AH-doh MOO-kah shvon-AHS-anna]

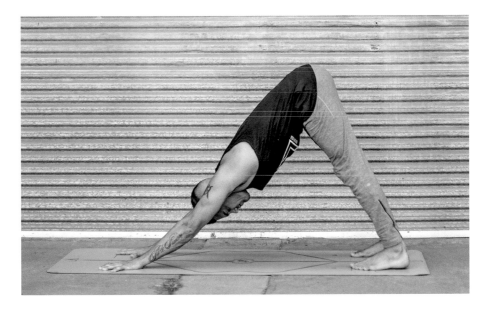

This pose is a great way to stretch and open the body, and once learned, it will give you a familiar posture to come back to regularly throughout your practice.

Five points of focus

1. Place your hands and feet shoulder- and hip-width apart as you create a triangle shape in the body.
2. Ground the balls of your feet into the mat, allowing your heels to rest comfortably (but they do not need to touch the floor).
3. Press the hands and palms firmly in the mat with the pressure mainly on the thumb and first finger side of the hand.
4. Rotate your pelvis and tailbone towards the sky by tilting the sit bones upward and spiralling your thighs inward and back.
5. Keep a long line in the spine, trying not to let the belly drop towards the floor.

73

FIERCE POSE

Utkatasana *(OOT-kah-TAHS-anna)*

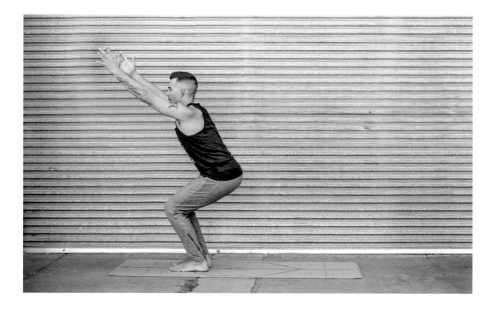

This is often referred to as Chair pose because of the shape that is made in the body.

Five points of focus

1. From Tadasana (Mountain pose), bend the knees and sink the hips, creating a chair-like shape, keeping the weight of the body grounded through the heels.
2. Create support with internal (medial) rotation of the thighs.
3. Lengthen the tailbone so the spine is long.
4. The upper body creates a 45-degree angle extending the torso away from the hips.
5. Reach the hands to the sky, broadening the back through external (lateral) rotation of the biceps.

WARRIOR ONE

Virabhadrasana I *[veer-ah-bah-DRAHS-anna]*

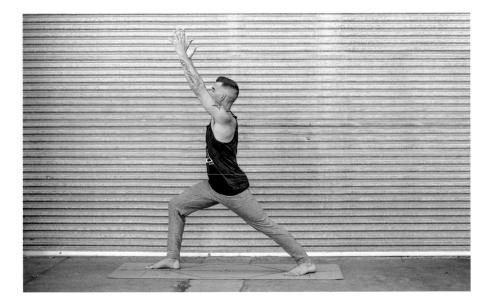

The aim of the pose is to keep the hips in a closed position.

Five points of focus

1. Stand with your back foot at 45 degrees with the weight on the outside edge of the foot and the knee tracking the same line as the ankle.
2. The front foot is evenly placed with the knee tracking the same line as the ankle, feet slightly narrower than hip width.
3. Square the hips forward by drawing the back hip forward, creating internal (medial) rotation of the thigh.
4. Elevate the spine (think Tadasana – Mountain pose).
5. Extend the fingers to the sky without creating an arch through the spine.

WARRIOR TWO

VIRABHADRASANA II *(veer-ah-bah-DRAHS-anna)*

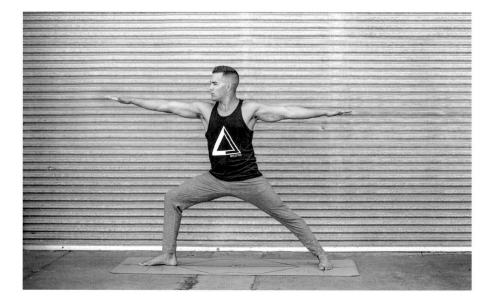

The aim of the pose is to keep the hips in an open position.

Five points of focus

1. Stand with your back foot at 45 degrees with the weight on the outside edge of the foot and the knee tracking the same line as the ankle.
2. The front foot is evenly placed with the knee tracking the same line as the ankle and external (lateral) rotation of the thigh.
3. The hips are in an open position, allowing the back hip to find a comfortable angle slightly pointing forward.
4. Elevate the torso parallel to the long side of the mat and extend each arm, front and back.
5. Turn the head forward, looking down the middle finger of your front hand.

GARLAND POSE

Malasana *[mal-AHS-anna]*

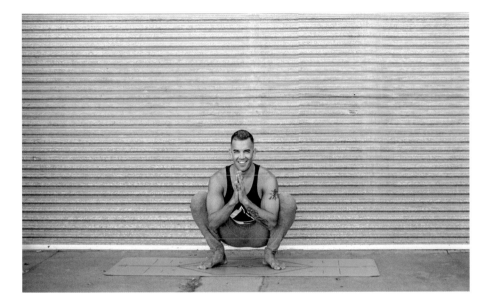

This pose is all about opening you up gently and carefully. It is also how many Easterners will naturally sit and eat or use the bathroom.

Five points of focus

1. Start with the feet hip-width apart and turned out at 45 degrees.
2. Bend the knees and come into a squat position, sinking the hips towards the floor (note, your heels don't have to touch the ground).
3. Rest the triceps on the knees or inner thighs.
4. Bring the hands to the centre of the chest to create a steady connection.
5. Lift the chest up as you draw the shoulders down the back; don't hunch.

HALF-MOON POSE

Ardha Chandrasana *[ARE-dah chan-DRAHS-anna]*

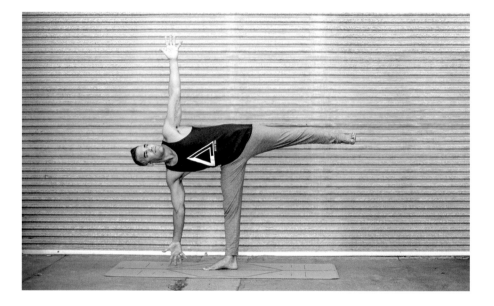

The most challenging part of this pose is finding balance.

Five points of focus
1. Start with the standing leg strong and pointing forward, in line with the knee.
2. Lift the back leg parallel off the ground, lengthening and extending to the back of the room while keeping the foot engaged.
3. Use the bottom hand for support on the ground or on a block.
4. Open and stack the hips as you lift up from the standing leg.
5. Reach the top hand to the sky as you extend the head and neck long.

EAGLE POSE

Garudasana *(gah-roo-DAHS-anna)*

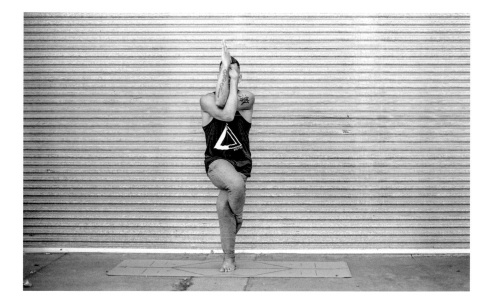

This pose is great to rinse and cleanse the internal organs, the digestion, the reproductive organs and to help circulation.

Five points of focus

1. Start from standing; shift your weight onto one standing leg.
2. Lower the hip and bend the knee of the raised leg and cross it over the top of the standing thigh.
3. On the same side of the body as the raised leg, wrap the arm under the opposite arm, creating a bind.
4. Lift the elbows to the same height as the shoulders, while drawing the shoulders down the back to make space.
5. Keep your eyes steady on one point to find balance.

DANCER POSE

Natarajasana *[nat-ah-raj-AHS-anna]*

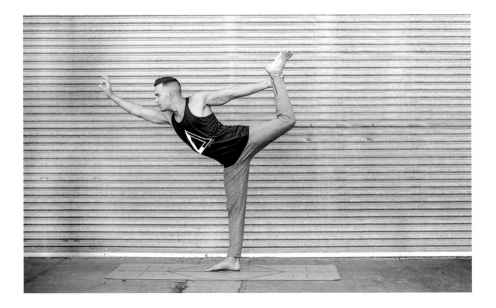

And they say guys can't dance. Be graceful – this pose is about the balance of reaching forward and kicking back.

Five points of focus

1. Start from standing; shift your weight onto one standing leg.
2. Bend the knee of your raised leg and grab the foot from the inside or outside, creating a bind.
3. Reach up with the opposite hand and start to shift the weight forward.
4. Reach forward with the front hand as you kick the raised leg back into your hand, creating even weight distribution for balance, but do not open or stack the hips.
5. Keep the shoulders away from the ears, and feel the stretch in the raised leg.

TREE POSE

Vriksasana [vrik-SHAS-anna]

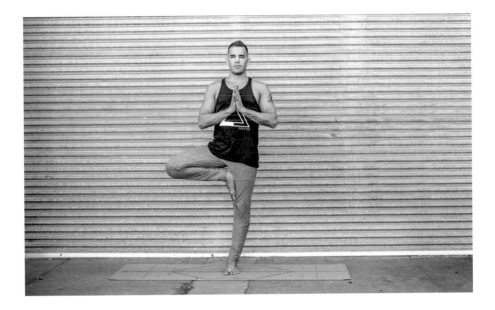

Yup, that pose – the most recognisable yoga pose in the world.

Five points of focus

1. Start from standing; shift your weight onto one standing leg.
2. Elevate your other leg and place the sole of the foot above or below the knee on the inside of the standing leg.
3. Keep an external (lateral) rotation in the lifted thigh.
4. Create length in the spine by keeping an upward lift in the chest.
5. Use different variations of the arms to create challenge.

TRIANGLE POSE

Trikonasana *(trik-cone-AHS-anna)*

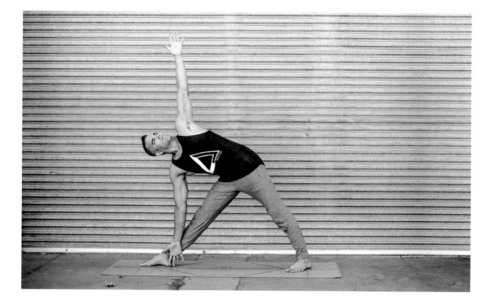

This pose is notoriously tricky. The key is to place your bottom hand wherever is comfortable and remember – yoga is for everyone, but not every pose has to be!

Five points of focus

1. From a Warrior Two shape (see page 76), straighten your front leg, lifting up from the hip.
2. Keeping a tilt in the pelvis, lengthen the torso forward to create space in the spine.
3. Let the bottom hand come to rest in any comfortable position, on a block or the floor.
4. Keep a connection to the floor with the back foot, turned out at 45 degrees.
5. Reach your top hand up, and keep the crown of the head in line with the neck and spine.

BOW POSE

Dhanurasana *(dan-oor-AHS-anna)*

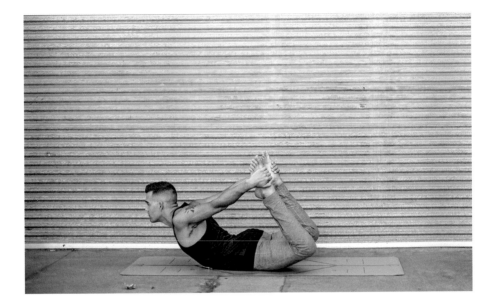

This pose is about moving and protecting the spine. Make sure you're gentle. The aim isn't to see how high you can lift off the ground, but about opening the chest.

Five points of focus

1. Starting face-down on the mat, bend the knees and grab the feet from the outside.
2. Ensure the knees are only hip-width apart, and begin to kick back into the hands as you lift the chest off the mat.
3. Keeping the shoulders drawing down the back, lift the chest to a comfortable height.
4. Keep the head in line with the neck and spine.
5. Only go to the point that is comfortable.

BRIDGE POSE

Setu Bandhasana *[SAY-too ban-DAHS-anna]*

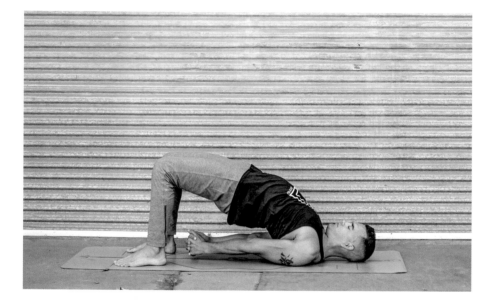

This is a safe way to prepare for Wheel pose; it's important to always ensure you're warming the spine before taking it into deeper backbending.

Five points of focus

1. Start on your back with knees bent and feet hip-width apart and parallel on the floor.
2. Start by lifting the hips as you press back into the mat, bringing them to the same height as the knees.
3. Engage the thighs with an internal (medial) rotation, creating space across the lower back.
4. Interlace your fingers behind your back and walk the shoulder blades together for grounded support.
5. For safety in the neck, don't look around and keep space between the neck and the mat.

WHEEL POSE

Urdhva Dhanurasana
[oord-vah dan-oor-AHS-anna]

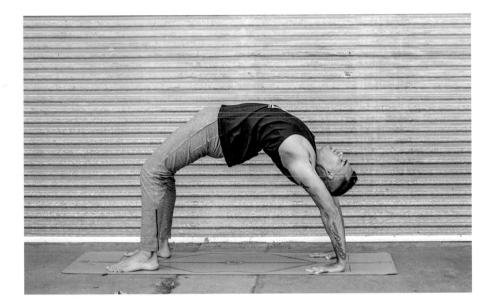

This pose will tempt you not to breathe; ensure that you keep a steady breath when practising this pose.

Five points of focus

1. Start on your back with knees bent and feet hip-width apart and parallel on the floor.
2. Place the hands above the head on the mat behind you, shoulder-width apart, with the fingers facing in the direction of your feet.
3. Engage the thighs with an internal (medial) rotation, creating space across the lower back.
4. Keep the elbows shoulder-width apart and, in one sweeping motion, press through the hands and feet and rise up.
5. Keep the head and neck in line with the natural curve of your spine.

BOAT POSE

Navasana *[nah-VAHS-anna]*

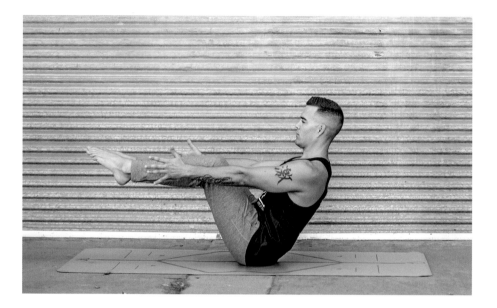

The focus of this pose is the lift and length of the chest, not how high you can get your legs.

Five points of focus

1. Sit on the floor with your knees bent and chest in an elevated position.
2. Extend the arms and fingers forward, creating balance.
3. Lift the heels from the mat together, so that the calves are parallel to the ground to steady the body without letting the chest drop back.
4. Engage the core, pulling navel to spine, to support the pose.
5. Activate the pose further by extending the legs without letting the chest drop back (advanced variation).

HALF PIGEON POSE

Eka Pada Rajakapotasana I
[EK-kah PAH-dah RAH-jah-capo-TAHS-anna]

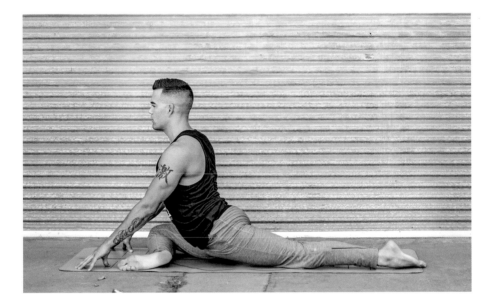

Approach this pose with caution if you have knee injuries or sensitivities.

Five points of focus
1. Start from a Downward-facing Dog (see page 73); bring one leg forward and place it parallel to the front edge of the mat with the toes flexed.
2. Release the back leg, knee and foot to the mat to create a line of connection to the floor.
3. Draw the front hip back to square the hips to the front.
4. Using your hands, elevate the chest and find length in the spine.
5. To deepen the pose, release the torso onto the elbows or chest.

SEATED FORWARD FOLD

Paschimottanasana
[PAS-chee-moh-tan-AHS-anna]

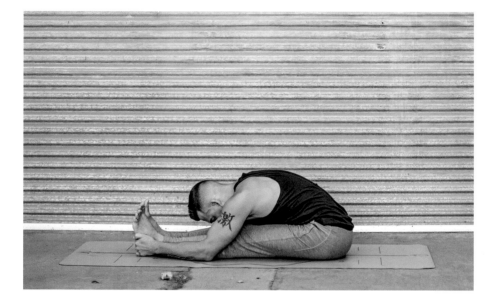

When seated, this pose stretches the full back line of the body.

Five points of focus
1. From a seated position, extend the legs forward, starting with a bend in the knees.
2. Before you reach forward reach up, extending the arms, spine and torso to create space.
3. Bend forward, grabbing the outsides of the feet and allowing the chest to fall forward in extension.
4. Keep the knees bent as much as you need to reach the feet.
5. Draw the shoulders down the back, creating space around the ears as you draw your chest to your thighs, not nose to toes.

CORPSE POSE

Savasana *[shav-AHS-anna]*

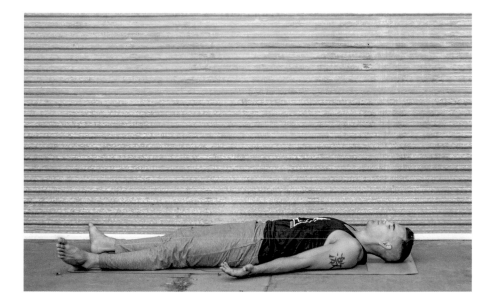

The best-loved yoga pose, the final rest taken at the end of a class.

Five points of focus

1. Lie down gently on your back.
2. Let the eyes close, palms face up, toes fall outward.
3. Release any tension or distraction from the body.
4. Allow the body to be at ease.
5. This is the ultimate pose in any yoga class: it is never optional (but why would you even ask?).

Now you know enough to get going. Take as much time as you need to learn the above poses. Try them out at home and then get to a class and put them into practice.

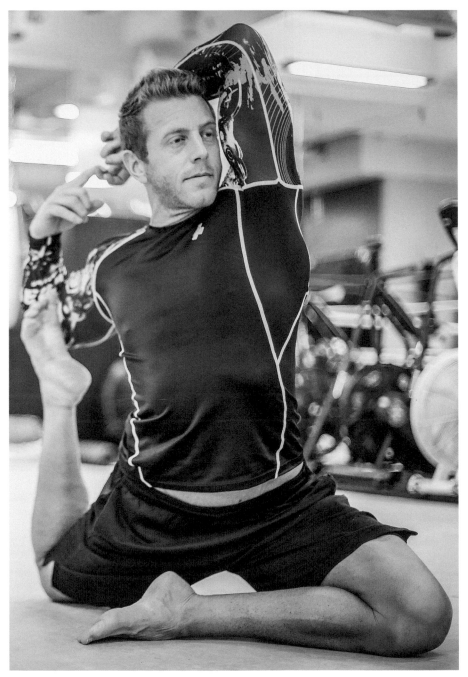

Darrel Erxleben

'EVERY PERSON'S POSTURES WILL LOOK AND FEEL DIFFERENT. THERE IS NO RIGHT OR WRONG'

But Am I Doing It Right?

Well, you're not doing it wrong, but you might be doing it differently. And that's what yoga is all about. In yoga the poses need to be aligned safely in a natural range of motion that reflects your body (and body type). And whether you realise it or not, these poses will look different for everyone. Every person's strength, flexibility and mobility are different, and so every person's postures will look and feel different too. There is no right or wrong, just a matter of safety and respect for yourself.

Trying to make your yoga poses look like someone else's is like comparing apples to oranges. There is no point. At the end of the day, if it looks good, that's just your opinion.

But if it feels good, then you're doing it right.

Saluting the Sun
A basic warm-up suitable for everyone

Now that you understand some of the basic poses, the next step is to learn how they flow together. There are many styles of yoga; you may have heard of Hatha, Vinyasa, Yin, Restorative, Iyengar, Bikram, etc. But to make it simpler, let's talk about a style called

Vinyasa, a derivative of Ashtanga yoga and one of the most commonly found styles in Western yoga studios. In Vinyasa the teacher will link the poses with the breath, allowing you to connect it all together as you flow from one pose to the next.

At the start of these classes you will often practise a series of poses called sun salutations (surya namaskar) – a sequence that brings the body into mindful movement and honours the tradition of saluting the sun as it rises (see pages 94–97). Before starting any physical practice, however, it's important to warm the body and spine gently – this integration sequence is a great way to flex the spine and prepare the body for moving more actively.

1. Child's Pose
p. 65

2. Table-top Pose

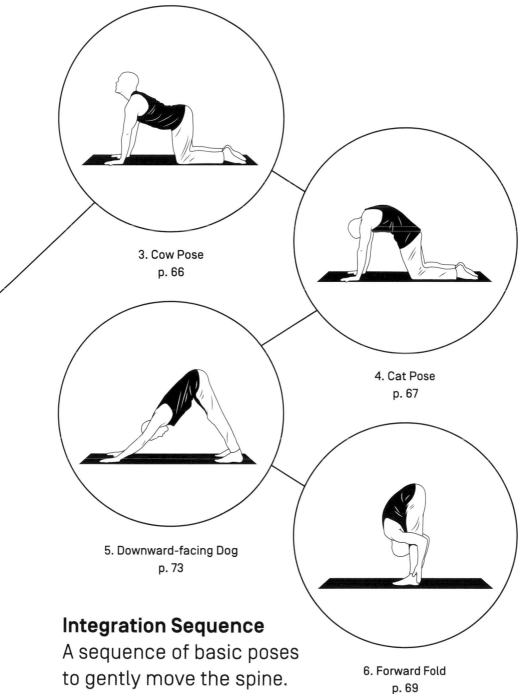

3. Cow Pose
p. 66

4. Cat Pose
p. 67

5. Downward-facing Dog
p. 73

6. Forward Fold
p. 69

Integration Sequence
A sequence of basic poses
to gently move the spine.

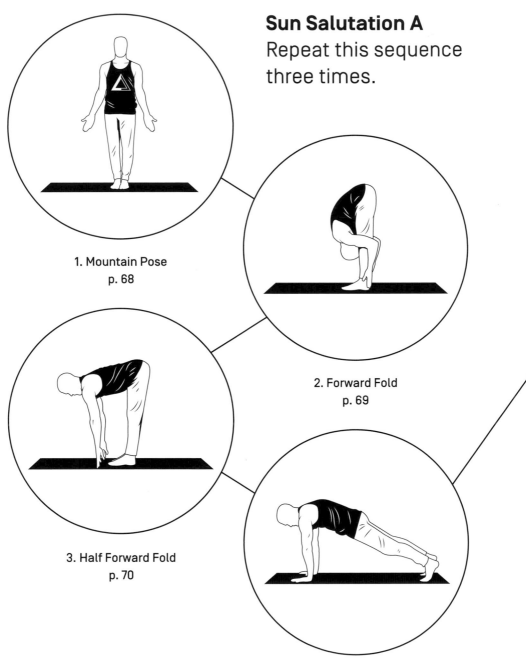

Sun Salutation A
Repeat this sequence three times.

1. Mountain Pose
p. 68

2. Forward Fold
p. 69

3. Half Forward Fold
p. 70

4. High Plank

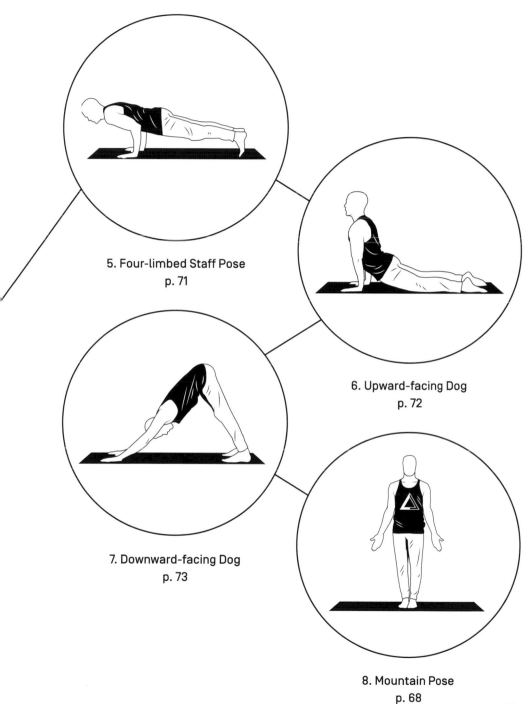

5. Four-limbed Staff Pose
p. 71

6. Upward-facing Dog
p. 72

7. Downward-facing Dog
p. 73

8. Mountain Pose
p. 68

Sun Salutation B

Sun salutations A and B are usually practised sequentially, one after the other. Try three rounds of A, followed by three rounds of B. It's a great way to start your day.

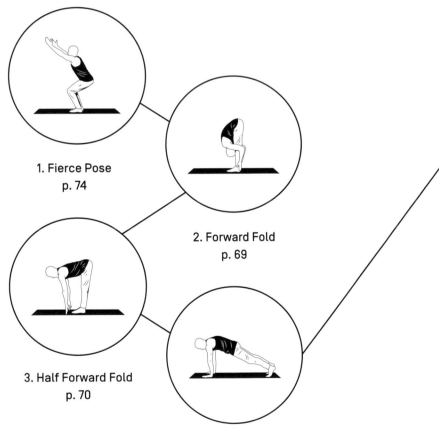

1. Fierce Pose
p. 74

2. Forward Fold
p. 69

3. Half Forward Fold
p. 70

4. High Plank

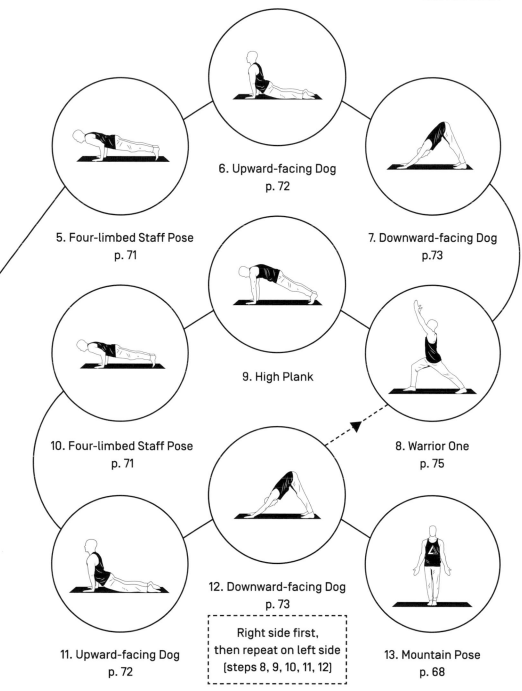

5. Four-limbed Staff Pose
p. 71

6. Upward-facing Dog
p. 72

7. Downward-facing Dog
p.73

9. High Plank

10. Four-limbed Staff Pose
p. 71

8. Warrior One
p. 75

12. Downward-facing Dog
p. 73

Right side first,
then repeat on left side
(steps 8, 9, 10, 11, 12)

11. Upward-facing Dog
p. 72

13. Mountain Pose
p. 68

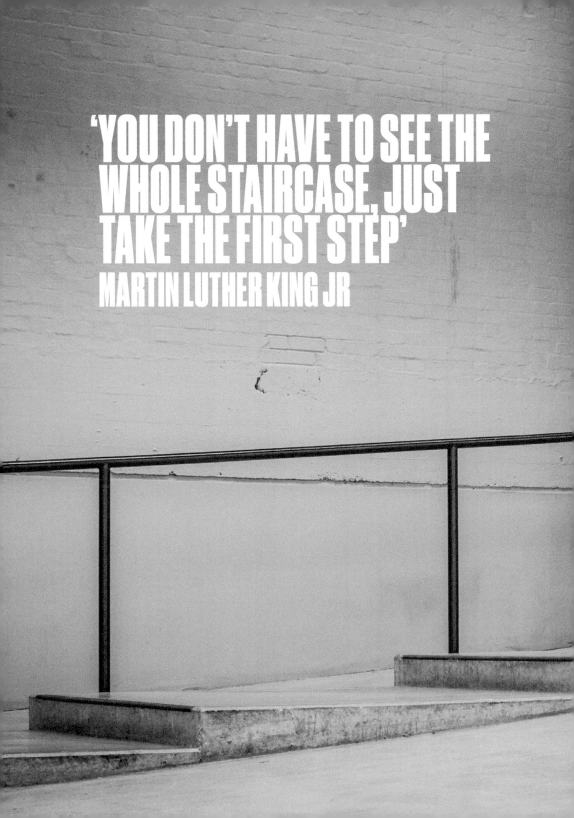

'YOU DON'T HAVE TO SEE THE WHOLE STAIRCASE, JUST TAKE THE FIRST STEP'
MARTIN LUTHER KING JR

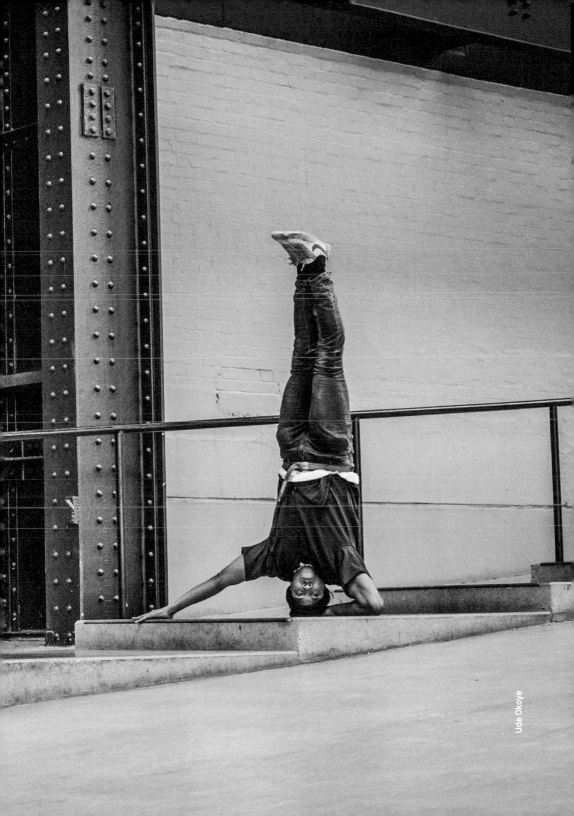

MEET THE BOYS
NICHOLAS HIGGINS
LONDON

What's your story? I went to school in Somerset, England, and went off travelling as soon as I hit 18. I love skiing, so I got a job as a ski instructor in Switzerland. It was such a cool job, but it took a toll on my body: too much après ski. It also got pretty claustrophobic in such a small place; there wasn't much room to breathe.

What's the worst job you've ever had? Man, I've had so many. I've been a dishwasher, worked in a garden centre for £2.50 an hour, been a granite-polisher, worked as a runner on music videos where you're up all night in the freezing cold, unpaid, for the privilege of 'putting the artist's name on your CV'. The hardest was working with a company who had a stage at music festivals in the UK. I was behind the bar serving hundreds and hundreds of people who were all having far too much fun.

What is one fact that most other people wouldn't know about you? I'm terrified of space. Outer, not personal.

What's the biggest challenge in being a guy who practises yoga? It still happens sometimes that other guys' reflex reaction to my telling them what I do is laughter! But it's rarer these days, and it's amazing to see more and more guys trying it out and loving it.

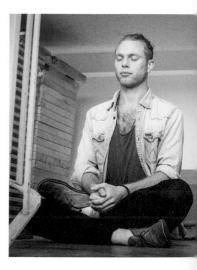

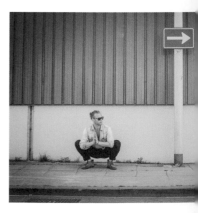

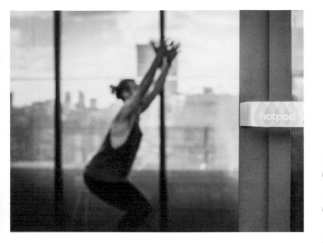

SHOULDER STANDER.
STUDIO OWNER.
SKI INSTRUCTOR.
YOGI.

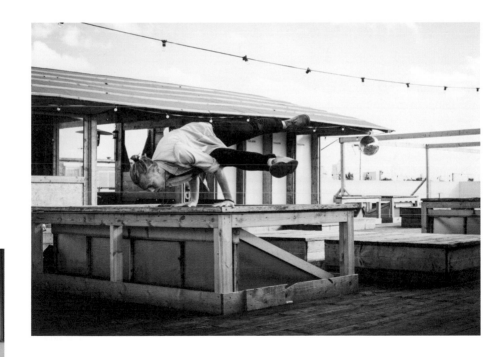

@hotpodyoga
Read more at boysofyoga.com
@boysofyoga

MEET THE BOYS
JONAS PINZKE
STOCKHOLM

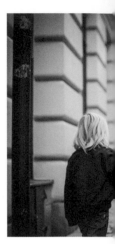

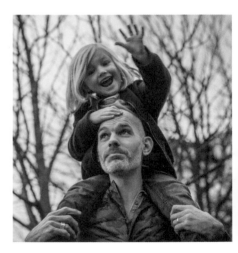

What's your story? I grew up in a socialist ghetto with academics and political immigrants from all over the world. My parents were true idealists and I sat on my father's shoulders at every political demonstration during the 70s. Now, having just turned 40 and looking back, I realise that this formed my life in more ways than I can (or sometimes want to) believe. I can see now that all political views can be dogmatic and narrow-minded. The rebel in me meant I had to challenge my parents' beliefs to become a 'successful' art director working in advertising. But on the other hand, I believe that I have gained a solid foundation in understanding and believing in the equality of every human (and animal!), everywhere.

Now I'm a father of two children, which I guess defines me more than most other things. It might be a cliché but oh-so true. These two minions are my yoga today. Challenging me, grounding me, making me unconditionally me.

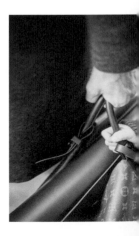

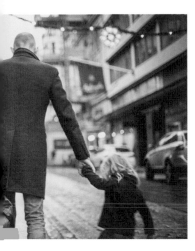

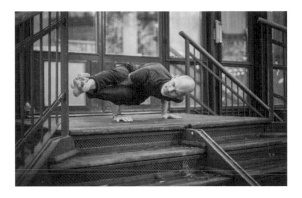

TRUE GENTLEMAN.
STYLE ICON.
CREATIVE DIRECTOR.
YOGI.

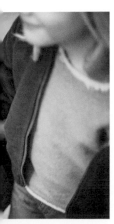

What advice would you give to someone stepping onto the mat for the first time? You are not the first and you are not alone. We have all been there. We have all felt the insecurity and the inadequacy. Just do it, and do it again and again. I know a smart dude who once wrote 'some guys think that yoga makes you less of a man, the truth is it makes you a better one'...

When was the last time you cried? A few weeks ago I realised that my kids will eventually grow up. It just became clear to me that at a certain point they won't need me any more. I was crying because it was both beautiful and terrifying at the same time.

What is your favourite quote or personal mantra? 'Okah samastah sukhino bhavantu.' May all beings everywhere be happy and free.

I hope that my thoughts, words and actions in some way contribute to that happiness and freedom for all.

@coolhead.warmheart
Read more at boysofyoga.com
@boysofyoga

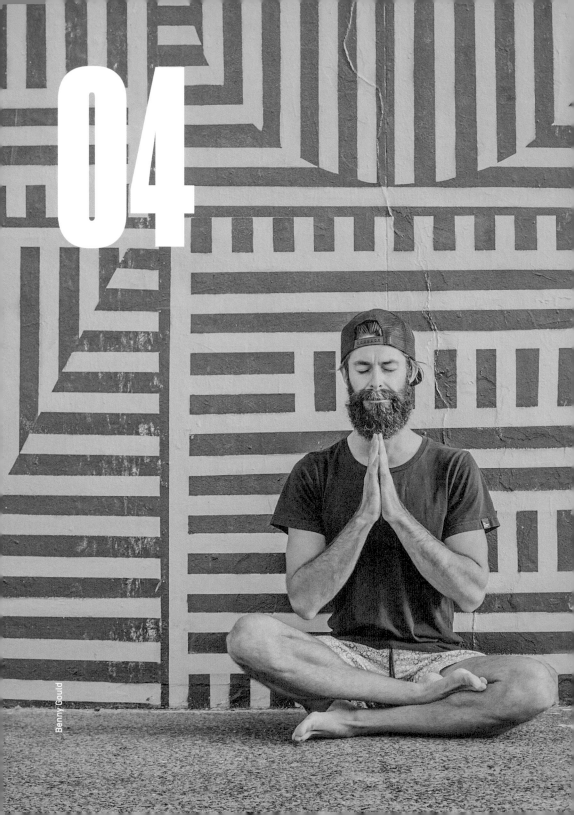

04

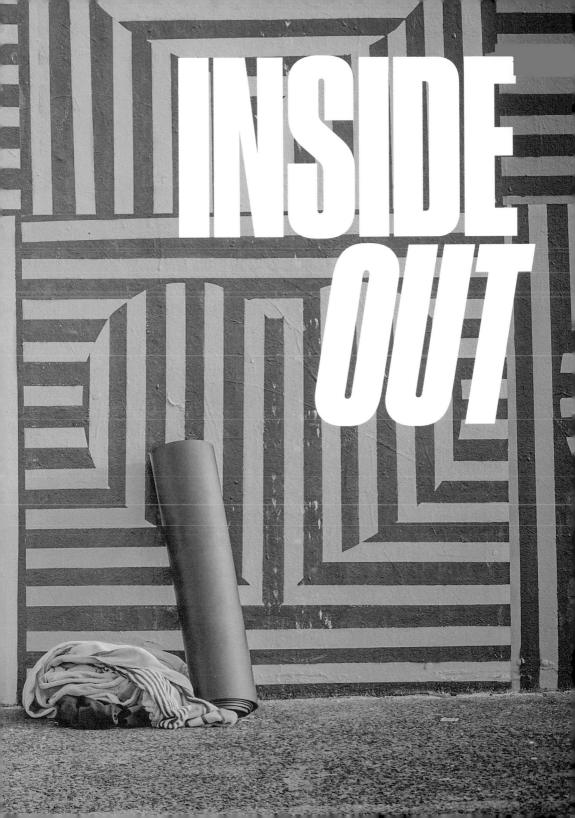

It's Not A Work Out,
It's A Work In

Now that you know more about the
physical aspect, it's time to look
inward. The true power of yoga is
what it does for us on the inside,
enabling us to create a connection
with ourselves, each other and the
world around us. It's why we need to
remember that yoga is a work in, not
just work out.

   Ultimately, the practice provides
space: in the mind and body and
in your everyday life. Yoga helps to
calm the chaos and, when practised
authentically, we can live from the
inside out.

But, Sometimes We Must Sweat Before We Surrender

It was simple: go to yoga, move, sweat, feel great, repeat. This was how I started, and for many other people this is how it begins too.

The physical practice of yoga is one of the best ways to start because it's tangible. We can feel and see the benefits in our daily lives straight away. It is a great preparation for the inside work, so it should never be devalued. In yoga, we move the body to narrow our focus and ultimately prepare for sitting in stillness. How long and how much movement we need is personal and differs from day to day.

What I remember most about starting yoga was how much I enjoyed the physical element. It made me move, sweat and feel good. It was something I could understand and see immediate value in, even though I felt I wasn't very good at it. It kept me coming back.

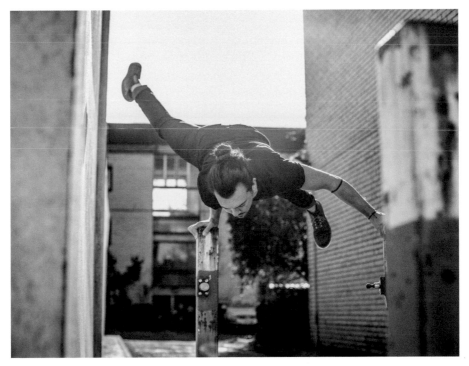

Jake Paul White

It's What's On The Inside

Yoga has a way of stirring up what's on the inside. It brings everything to our attention. The physical practice is the doorway inside to the things that we can't often see or don't want to address. By moving the body through a sequence of poses, we set the scene for the internal work to happen. It's never easy to look within, to acknowledge, 'Yeah, I'm a person that gets easily annoyed,' or, 'I'm stuck living in the past, it's time to move on' or, 'This relationship is not working'. There is huge value in knowing and it gives us the awareness and opportunity to grow.

There is so much within us that can't be seen: thoughts, emotions, anxieties and fears; internal tightness, aches and pains and real vulnerabilities. We're always dealing with something. Practising yoga on and off the mat helps to cultivate an inward attitude. In life, it's easy to ignore the things we can't see. We all tend to focus on the things that are right in front of us rather than the things within us.

So when practising yoga, stop worrying what the shape is supposed to look like and focus on what is going on at a deeper level.

Let's break it down.

Take Chair pose, or utkatasana. Have you practised this pose before? For me, this is anything but fun. It conjures up feelings and emotions like anger, frustration, anxiety, obligation, fear.

Anger because I don't actually want to be there.

Frustration because I don't know how long I'm going to be there.

Anxiety because I don't know how long I can stay there.

Obligation because I feel I have to be there.

Fear because I don't want to look bad if I can't hold the pose for as long as everyone else.

Yoga has a way of stirring things up on the inside. It brings everything to our attention and we can either address or ignore them.

ANGER because you don't actually want to be there.

Why are you angry? No one is forcing you to be in the pose. Anger has a way of misrepresenting reality, making us believe that this 'was done to us', rather than 'it's something we don't want to do'. We all get angry, it's true, but it's less about being angry, and more about acknowledging the reason why you are angry and how it's affecting you.

In yoga you can always do less; it's always allowed.

FRUSTRATION because you don't know how long you're going to be there.

For some people, Chair pose may not be an issue. In fact, the pose itself can be quite therapeutic, not to mention the incredible benefits it has for the body. But what frustrates you is that you never know how long you're going to be there for.

Some teachers will tell you and others won't, but stepping into the unknown is where the real yoga begins.

In yoga, like life, we can't control everything. We don't have all the answers and we cannot predict the future. Are you the type that gets annoyed when it rains unannounced or when you get caught at a red traffic light? Like it or not, this is how life works sometimes. We have no idea how long things are going to take, so stop worrying about it.

ANXIETY because you don't know how long you can stay there.

Anxiety often stems from doubt. Doubt that you're not good enough, that you look bad or that you can't live up to other people's expectations.

For me, my antidote to anxiety is simple: stop caring.

You don't owe anyone an explanation for the way you want to live your life.

'YOGA HAS A WAY OF STIRRING THINGS UP ON THE INSIDE. IT BRINGS EVERYTHING TO OUR ATTENTION'

OBLIGATION because you feel you have to be there.

Who do you feel obligated to? The teacher? The other students in the room? Yourself?

Allow me to let you in on a secret. As a yoga teacher who has been teaching for the better part of a decade, I still, to this day, don't care what my students do on the mat. Literally don't care (as long as it's not injurious). You can come and take a nap for an hour, you can practise every pose offered or you can do all the modifications and make it as easy as possible. Why? Because it's your body, your practice, your day and your life. As teachers, our role is to draw the outline of the experience. As the student, you can colour it in however you like.

Obligation is a funny thing. We believe we owe things to people when we don't. At times we believe that someone will feel mad, sad or let down if we do or don't do things. But regardless of their reaction, someone else's actions are solely their own; it's not on you to carry the weight of their expectations. When you take a moment to think about it, it is absurd, especially in a yoga class, sacrificing what feels good, what your preferences are, purely because you feel it's expected of you.

The only person you're obligated to in life and practice is yourself. Be selfish (without negative intent) and make sure that everything you do on and off the mat works in your favour.

FEAR because you don't want to look bad if you can't hold the pose for as long as everyone else.

Take a moment to think about it from another point of view: how often do you care whether the person next to you in class is doing the pose? Rarely. And if you're a teacher, how often are you offended if your students take a rest and don't do the pose? Never.

So, in the end, yes, you're in a Chair pose, **but you don't have to be**. You don't know how long you're going to be there, **but who cares?** They don't know what you're working with and you don't owe them anything. If the people around you in class are looking for a perfect Chair pose, tell them to go to Ikea. Being unable to make your body into a shape that looks like a chair and hold it isn't going to lessen who you are, and being able to do it isn't going to make you any better.

Do what works for you and stay true to who you are. That's the real practice of yoga.

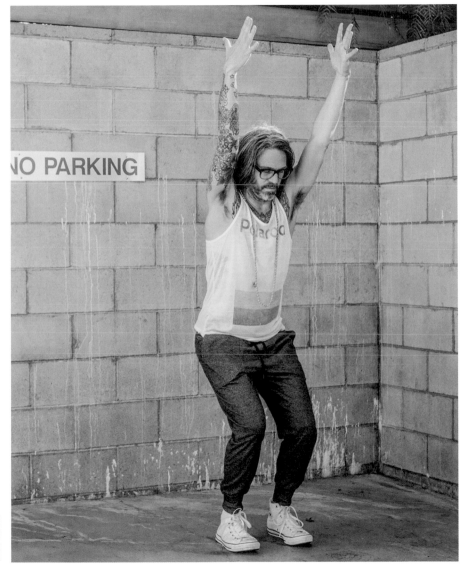

Chad Dennis

Take What You Need, Leave What You Don't

Have you ever been to an all-you-can-eat buffet, where there are piles and piles of delicious foods all around you? To my own certain demise, I go for everything. I pile on eight appetisers, ten different types of sides and as many mains as I can handle, and awkwardly waddle my way back to the table, balancing as many plates as I can.

Even though I know better, I always try to take everything, all at once.

Back at the table, I dive in. Everything gets shovelled into my mouth as fast as possible, but then it hits me – I'm full. In fact, I've already gone too far, and I'm only on the first course. I've got no room for anything else, let alone dessert, the best part. I'm defeated and I only just sat down.

And this is what can happen when we go to yoga: we try to do everything. Yoga is not a sprint, and you get no extra credit for doing it all. When we're first starting out, we can go too hard and try to do too much. We don't rest or take a Child's pose because we don't want to miss out, we think it's a sign of weakness, or worse, we feel we have an expectation to do everything. As humans, we have this internal sense of pride and ambition that tempts us to believe that we should always do more, rather than less. Maybe it's a cultural

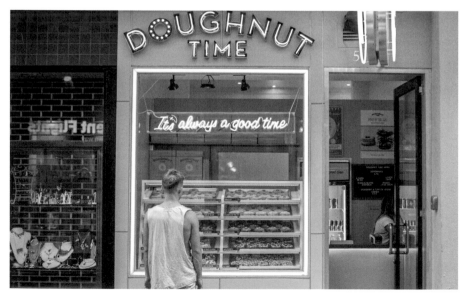

Duncan Parviainen

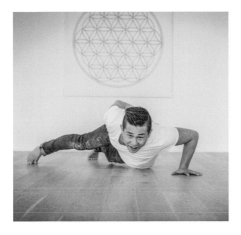

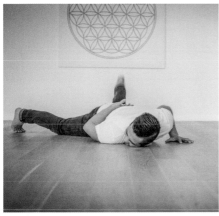

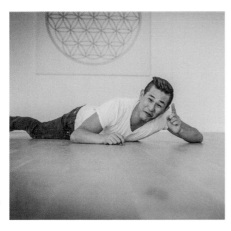

Jang-Ho Kim

thing. Maybe it's a guy thing. Maybe it's a YOU thing. Invest in rest and take it slow. Yoga isn't a competition, so don't make it one.

When you start to practise, know that there will be lots of opportunities and challenges on the mat throughout the class. We're offered the chance to try new poses, to do more, to explore advanced poses and modifications. But remember that you don't have to do everything. Less is more.

The real practice of yoga teaches us that the challenges we face in class are opportunities for us to pick and choose what's right in the moment; to simply take only the things that we absolutely need. Often, if you pile on too much and try to do everything at once, you'll miss out on the best parts.

Yoga is about enjoying the full experience. It's about knowing that in the course of a 60-minute class there will be highs and lows, fast and slow, strong and soft, so don't waste yourself on just the beginning. The power of the practice is the whole experience, from the first pose to the last. So make sure you start the class knowing this, do the class remembering it and finish the class appreciating it. Learn to take what you need and leave behind what you don't.

Just like the buffet, enjoy the whole meal, not all at once, but one bite at a time, and I guarantee you'll make it to dessert.

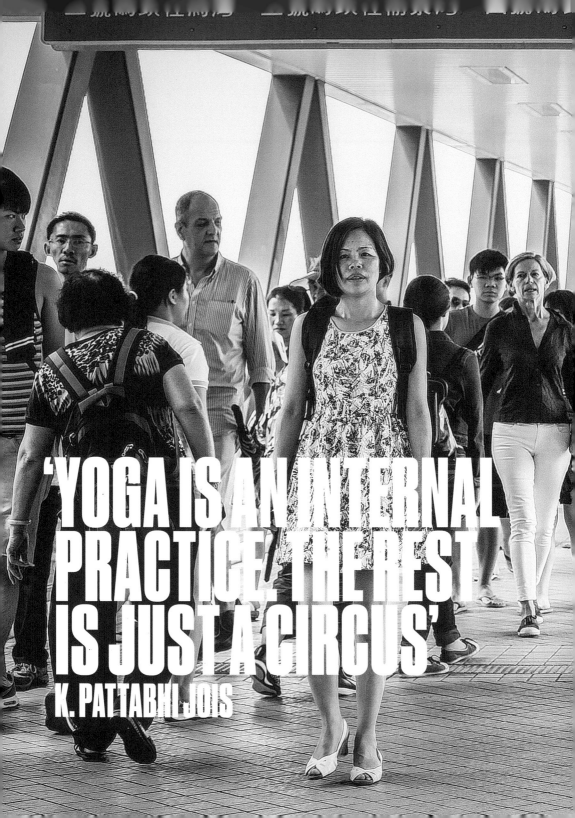

'YOGA IS AN INTERNAL
PRACTICE. THE REST
IS JUST A CIRCUS'
K. PATTABHI JOIS

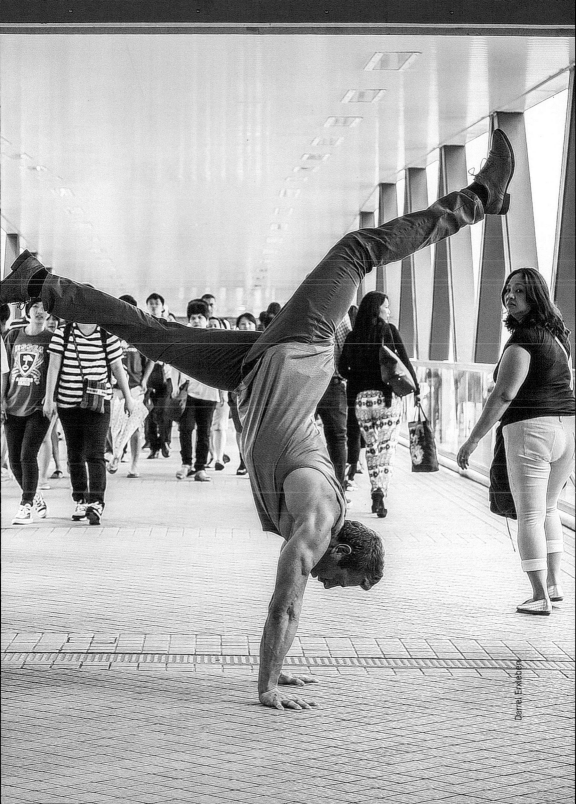

MEET THE BOYS

VICTOR CHAU

HONG KONG

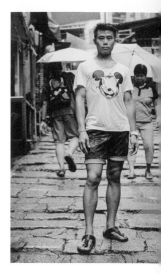

What's your story? Hong Kong born and bred, I was in media and luxury PR for a long time. Amid a crazy schedule, relentless industry gossip and way too much champagne, I found yoga a great way to help me focus. Honestly, I lived years and years of that party-hard, ego-driven lifestyle before I realised how little it all really meant. I had such a false sense of success then. I became more and more drawn to yoga to balance me. I began studying yogic philosophy and asking myself deeper questions. Eventually, I dedicated myself to a month of teacher training in India.

After living in Beijing for six years, I moved back to Hong Kong and now I live and breathe Hong Kong prana. I love teaching yoga to people from many backgrounds. In my mind, as long as you can move and breathe, you can do yoga.

It's fear that's stopping us from doing whatever we want to achieve. I get to watch people overcome that every day and it's a beautiful thing.

What is one fact that most other people wouldn't know about you? Most of my students and friends think that I eat super healthy. But I actually love fries and ice cream and I would have them every day if I could.

ADVENTURER. FRENCH-FRY ENTHUSIAST. NATURE JUNKIE. YOGI.

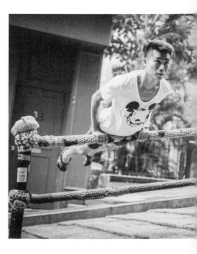

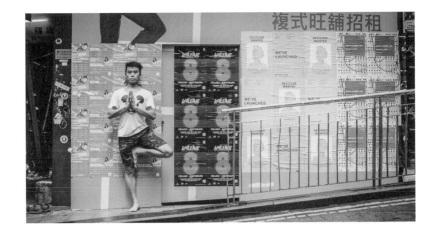

What was the biggest challenge when you first started? Finding my voice – literally. I first started teaching in Beijing and you really have to be able to teach in Mandarin if you want to get people to your classes. I was trained to teach in English, so having to teach in another language was tricky, to say the least!

Best yoga story? My 55-year-old student who did Crow pose for the first time ever – moments like that remind me why I want to keep teaching yoga for the rest of my life.

What's the biggest challenge in being a guy who practises yoga? It's really hard to convince other guys to practise yoga because they think they need to be really flexible. We easily fall into patterns of how we use and treat our bodies, and leaving that safety zone – trying yoga if you're a guy who's never been there before – can be hard. You don't need to be flexible – get on the mat!

Your mantra? Breathe deeply; you can always come back to Child's pose.

@victorchauyoga
Read more at boysofyoga.com @boysofyoga

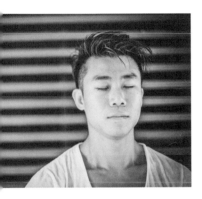

MEET THE BOYS
ADAM HUSLER
LONDON

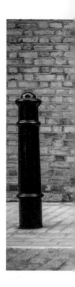

**BOXER.
ANATOMY GEEK.
WORKAHOLIC.
YOGI.**

How would you describe yourself? A mild workaholic, who's been lucky enough to turn work into something I love. The result is that despite little sleep, flights galore, a calendar that looks like conceptual art and an unreasonable amount of time multi-transport commuting around London, I'm still a very content guy. Meditation helps with that!

How would your mother describe you? A touch unpredictable, doesn't have an indoor voice and although she sometimes hides it, she's glad I didn't become a lawyer!

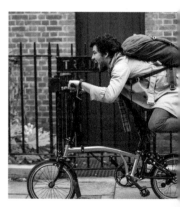

How did you get into yoga? As young guy, I spent the majority of my time on rugby pitches, in boxing rings, lifting metal plates and running marathons. Seemingly anything that involved internal stress, plenty of manliness, a liberal distribution of pain and constant knots and tension in my muscles and my mind. When I hit the working world with all of its stresses, I realised that I was spending a disproportionate amount of time with heavily tattooed men who enjoyed punching me. It was then I decided that stepping up my yoga practice could solve two problems. It would help me build

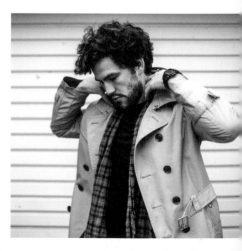

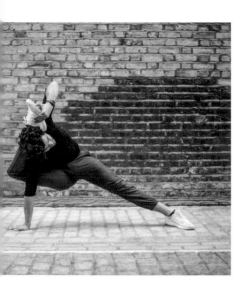

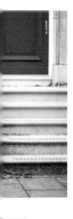

a social group that didn't want to watch *Rocky* re-runs or chat about workplace politics; and I could begin a little self-enquiry at a challenging time in my life, through a daily asana and meditation practice. The rest is history.

What keeps you coming back? From a teaching perspective, it's a privilege to be able to hold space and facilitate the chance for people to take a pause and begin to learn about themselves, initially at least, by controlling breath, body and mind though a physical asana experience. The more I teach the more I realise how little I know, and as someone who likes to know as much as I can and ask 'why' as much as a five-year-old, yoga and anatomy learning will keep me enjoying teaching for a long time to come.

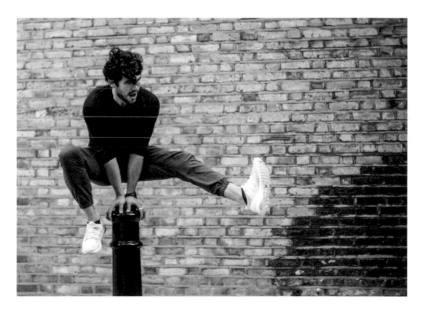

@adamhusler
Read more at boysofyoga.com @boysofyoga

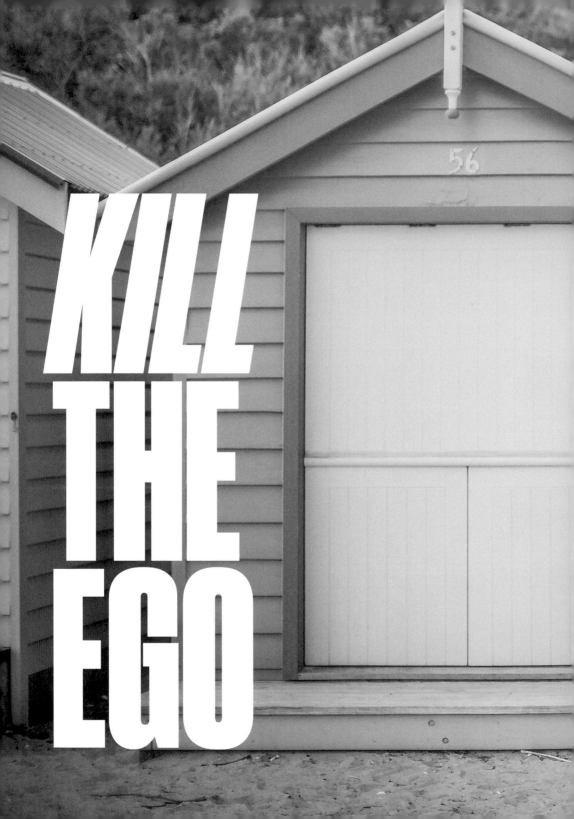

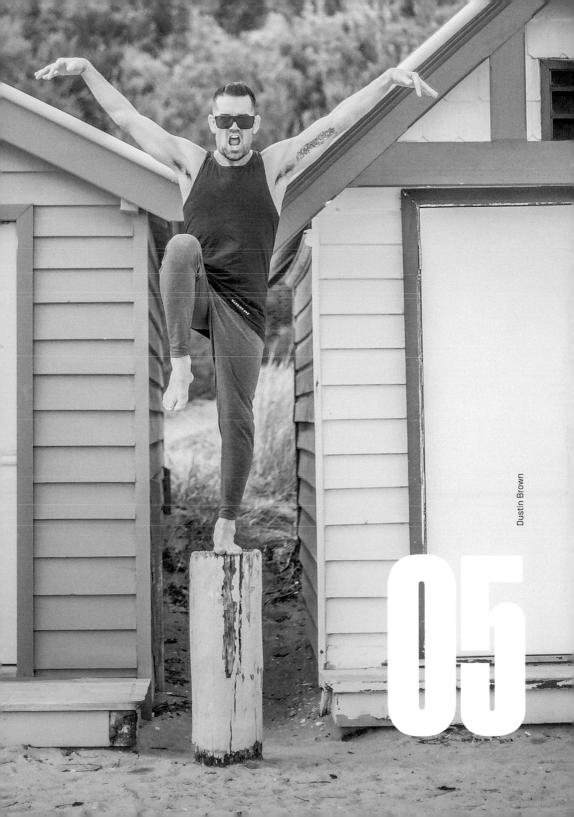

Dustin Brown

05

Kindness Has No Enemies

What is ego? We all have one, we all
know it's there, but what actually is
it? Is it that voice inside your head
telling you you're not good enough?
Or is it the voice warning you not
to do anything foolish or out of
character? Or is it just another
word for unwarranted pride and
over-confidence?

For me, it's all these things and more. Ego is the devil sitting on our shoulder, telling us that if we're not winning, then no one else should be. We all know this dance. Everyone has an ego, some bigger than others, some willing to admit it more than others, but it's always there, talking to us, tempting us and trying to manipulate us.

Is that really the way to live?

Is that the kind of person we really want to be?

Too often we let our egos make decisions that don't represent who we really are. These choices have lost us friends, caused arguments, got us in fights, ended relationships – all outcomes that perhaps, in time, we have regretted. We've all been there.

Sometimes we say sorry, sometimes we don't. And sometimes sorry won't do and the damage is already done.

Does any of this sound familiar?

You are not your ego. In his book *The Power of Now* (a book I believe everyone should make the time to read once in their life) Eckhart Tolle says that 'the ego is a negative projection upon a situation to change or manipulate it to make the individual feel better about themselves'. Take a moment to let that settle in. This one sentence that I read almost ten years ago has stuck with me and helped shift my actions and attitudes away from my ego.

So how do we control the ego? Or better yet, how do we let it go? I believe the antithesis of the ego is absolute kindness. It's treating everyone and everything with unconditional positivity. This is by no means an easy task. Life can easily be made into a competition. Western society breeds it – in school to get the grade, in work to get the promotion and in sports to get the win, competition is inherent as a societal normality. Kill or be killed is a hunter-gatherer hangover many of us still abide by. But in a modern world, if we choose kindness to all, then there is no need for the ego to feel threatened. At school we can all excel; if someone else gets the job, it's likely it wasn't right for us anyway. When we are kind, we are positive in all our actions and intentions. We have no enemies and we are in competition with no one else.

Josh Blau

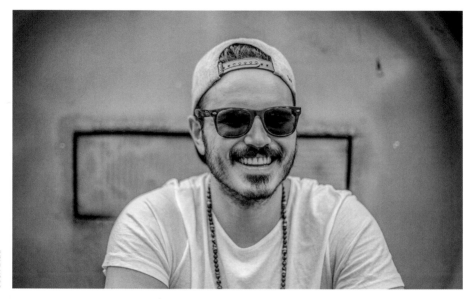

Live Inspired, Not Proud

For us to show pride, we must first have something to be proud of. It's a contextual emotion:

We are proud of our accomplishments because we have achieved them.

We are proud of our children because we have raised them.

We are proud of our heritage because it represents our history.

But these are all past accomplishments. No matter the situation, pride keeps referring us back. We cannot move forward with pride because it holds us back. It reminds us of what used to be, and through the ego we manipulate and defend our emotions if the current situation doesn't live up to past memories.

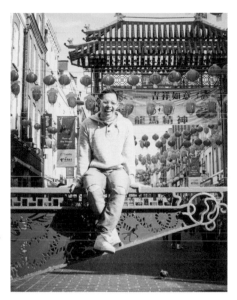

Jambo Truong

In Practice

Change your dialogue and notice how you use the word 'pride' (or proud). You'll be surprised how much it turns up in regular conversation.

'I'm so <u>proud</u> of you, son.'

'We should all be <u>proud</u> of the work we've done this week.'

'Show some <u>pride</u> for your team and how far they've come.'

These aren't offensive or negative phrases, but what would happen if these situations were threatened? This is when the ego would rear its ugly head.

Now, replace 'pride' with 'inspired'. This slight change in your wording will completely shift what you're saying. Pride celebrates the ego, while inspiration removes it.

'I'm <u>inspired</u> by you, son.'

'We should all be <u>inspired</u> by the work we've done this week.'

'We should be <u>inspired</u> by our team and how far they've come.'

Inspiration is inclusive and creates unity through positivity. Sometimes it's the smallest things that have the biggest effect on our whole outlook. I know it has changed my perspective, and I hope it does for you, too.

So instead of pride, change your perspective and word choice and move in a forward direction.

Live inspired, not proud.

I believe inspiration keeps us moving forward. The things that inspire us take our experiences from the past and bring them forward into the present and onward to the future. There is inspiration everywhere in life, and finding the positivity that takes us forward is always better than looking back into the past.

Fail More At Yoga

It's an innate human trait to want to not look stupid. It's in our DNA to defend the ego. I myself am guilty of liking to do things I'm good at, things I'm familiar with and things I've been successful at in the past. I have a sense of security in the certainty of the outcome. But when you don't try anything new, when you don't give yourself the chance to fail or fall down, you never learn anything new. You never grow.

In the practice, like life, there are times we don't try, not because we can't or don't want to, but because we're scared of what will happen if we fail. But the truth is failing is not a bad thing. For me, failing is simply trying something and not getting the outcome I planned for or wanted. But that doesn't mean it wasn't valuable and relevant. Often, fear is the biggest component.

We allow the mind to run through all the 'what-if' situations that may or may not happen and that inadvertently holds us back from that first attempt.

There is an old adage (I didn't make this up myself) that says to FAIL isn't a definite term; it's a continuous and ongoing process of learning.

To **FAIL** is your

First
Attempt
In
Learning

Every time you fail you learn something new.

One of my first yoga teachers, Duncan Peak from Power Living Yoga Australia, used to say, 'Don't be afraid to fail in a Crow pose; the truth is, the only thing that will get damaged is your ego, and that's ok.'

Remember this, and fail more at yoga.

'EVERY TIME YOU FAIL YOU LEARN SOMETHING NEW'

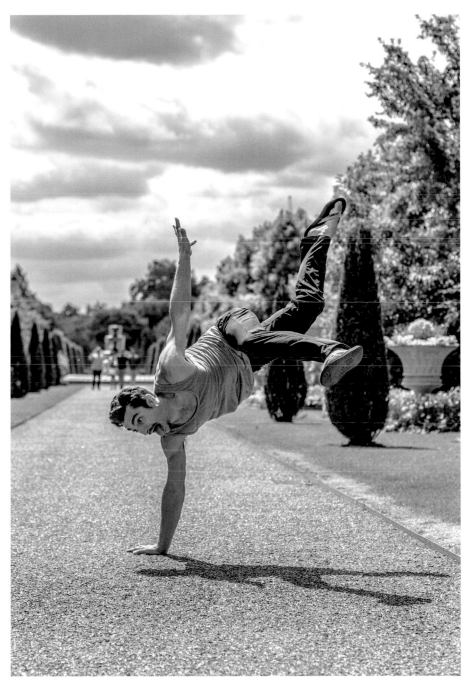

Matt Giordano

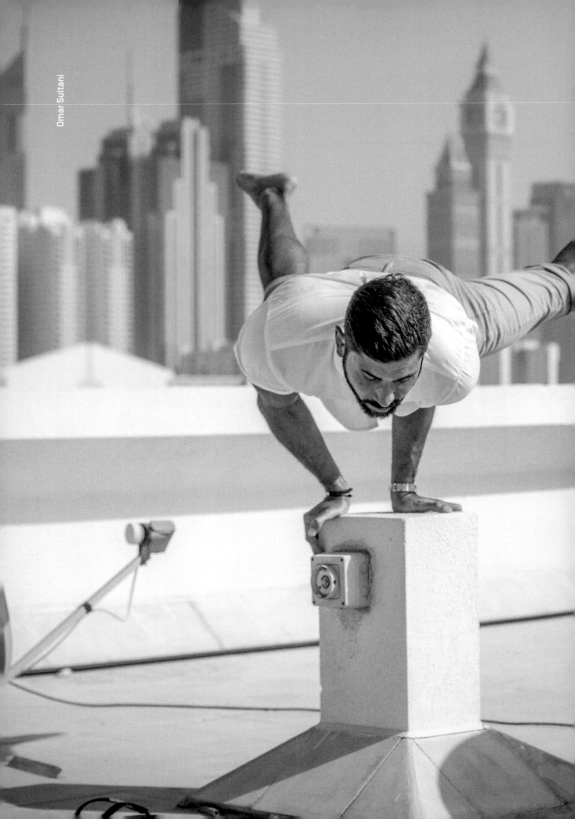

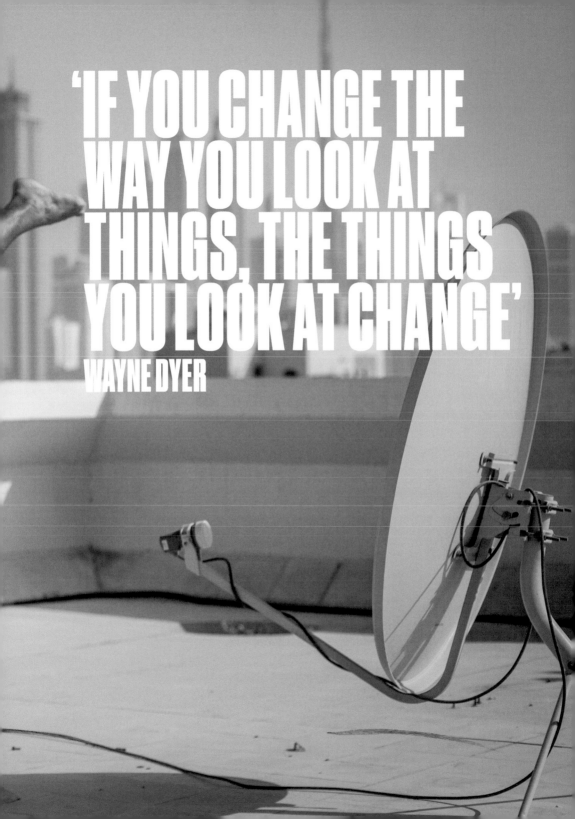

'IF YOU CHANGE THE WAY YOU LOOK AT THINGS, THE THINGS YOU LOOK AT CHANGE'

WAYNE DYER

MEET THE BOYS

MIKE AIDALA
NEW YORK

PADDLE BOARDER. OLYMPIC WEIGHTLIFTER. LOVE SEEKER. YOGI.

What's your story? I'm a lifelong athlete who grew up playing mainstream sports. I played football in college, then, when I graduated, I competed in SUP (stand-up paddle boarding), racing and Olympic weightlifting – not at the same time! But, to be honest, I soon became bored with the pressure to make faster times and lift heavier weights, and I was looking for something more – something that would engage my mind, body and soul. Yoga came to me, as it does for so many, at a transitional point in my life, and I fell in love with the journey inward.

How did you get into yoga? Being an athlete and trainer, I love the hard work and grind of working on myself physically. I became interested in yoga as a way to work on myself mentally and spiritually, while still being able to move.

My first class wasn't easy – I was moving my body in ways it had not had to move before. But that provided a whole different challenge – one that didn't involve personal bests or competition with everyone else in the room.

Yoga literally enhances our ability to experience life! That is so real and raw.

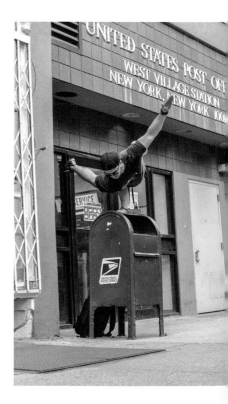

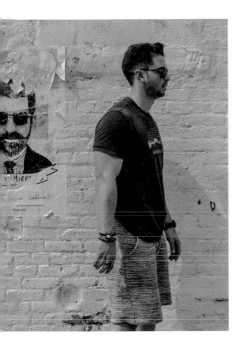

What was the biggest challenge when you first started? Confidence. Being 6ft 1in tall, weighing over 200lb and coming from a mainstream sports background I had to learn to accept myself real quick. This practice teaches you that kind of self-acceptance, physically and mentally, and I want to make sure guys know that it's for everyone – every body: male and female, small and large.

What's the biggest challenge in being a guy who practises yoga? Not being taken seriously. I learned early on that there are different teachers for different people and you can't please everybody. I don't know all the sutras or all the Sanskrit, but that's ok. I know plenty of other things and I focus on them. We all have plenty to offer.

Yoga is time for number one. It offers a space to go inside and be entirely selfish, but selfless at the same time.

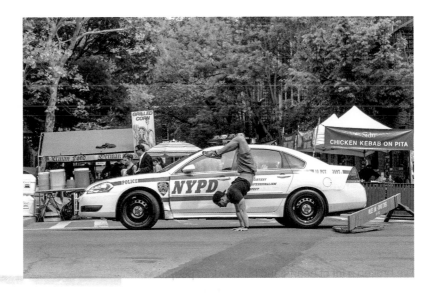

@mike.aidala
Read more at boysofyoga.com @boysofyoga

MEET THE BOYS
OCTAVIO SALVADO
BALI

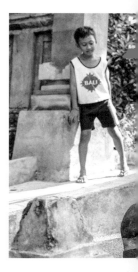

What's your story? I was born and raised in Melbourne, Australia. After ten years in India and Southeast Asia, I now call the Island of the Gods – Bali – home. As a teenager I studied psychology at university. They were the most boring years of my life. I knew there was a better way for me to serve my purpose. I just needed to find it. So, naturally, I went to India and I never went back home.

How would you describe yourself? Intense, passionate, difficult, confident, mildly arrogant, purpose-driven, capable, sunny and infectiously positive – when I'm in a good mood. When I'm not: some kind of raging dinosaur with sharp teeth and thumbs. And that's why I practise yoga.

Ever done anything you're not proud of? A lot. I'm a creature driven by purpose, like a red rag to a bull. My red rag is yoga. This seems like an inherently positive purpose, but I've often lost sight of the necessity to also nourish my personal relationships. I've broken a lot of hearts and hurt a lot of people with my single-mindedness. It's never intentional, but that's hardly the point. I'm not proud of that.

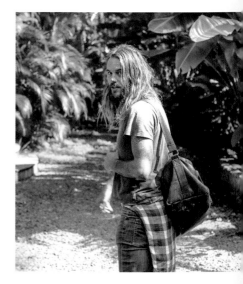

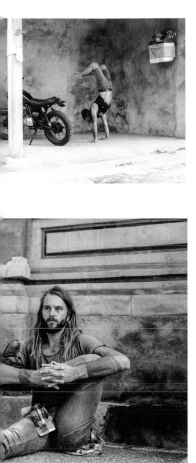

What's your favourite drink? Coffee and red wine. I can't tell you if I actually like these things or if I'm just rebelling against the stereotypes of what it means to be spiritual and yogic. Actually, that's a lie. I love coffee and red wine. Guilty.

Tell us a fact that other people don't know about you. Once I spent four hours teaching myself how to play 'Halo' by Beyoncé on the guitar. And I gotta say, I pretty much nailed it.

Have you faced many challenges along the way? Choosing this path has meant that I have had to sacrifice being close to my family. I put on a brave face, but it's very challenging, and always has been. Now that my dad is getting older and my nieces are growing up, I find my thoughts drifting to them a lot, and it's usually with a tinge of sadness in my heart.

Other than that ... being a stiff, white male has been pretty challenging – and I'm not talking about my hamstrings! I try to go to every backbend workshop on Bali – I call it 'ego management'. My mantra is 'Bridge pose is beautiful, Bridge pose is beautiful ...'

@octaviosalvado
Read more at boysofyoga.com
@boysofyoga

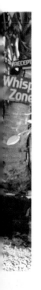

COFFEE DRINKER. TATTOO ENTHUSIAST. MOTORCYCLE COLLECTOR. YOGI.

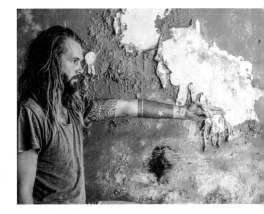

MEET THE BOYS
DUNCAN PARVIAINEN
TORONTO

What's your story? I grew up in a small town in Canada, where my family lived off the grid (our house was powered by a windmill and solar panels) in a ten-acre forest. I spent my summers canoe-tripping in northern Canada, building character as some would say: getting eaten alive by mosquitoes, tempting death on the rapids and being chewed up by nature. I became a canoe-tripping guide and led 10- to 17-year-olds on expeditions. It was tough but gratifying work.

We've all done a few things we aren't too proud of. Care to share one? I once stole eggs from a bird's nest when I was a young kid. I remember feeling bad about it, but I selfishly wanted to raise the eggs myself in my bedroom with hot-water bottles. My dream was to have my own bird family. I ended up dropping both eggs on the floor one day and felt like not only a thief, but also a murderer. (This might be the reason why I've been vegetarian for the last ten years.)

How did you get into yoga? I was talking to a friend and she said to me, 'Duncan, I think you would really like yoga. Come to one of my classes!' I attended her class and had NO idea what I was

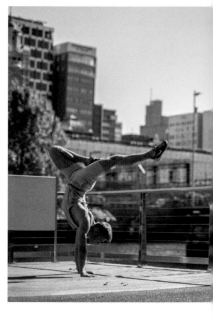

IRON MAN. CANOE GUIDE. PHILOSOPHER. YOGI.

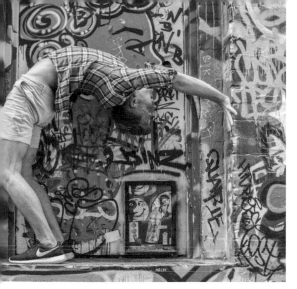

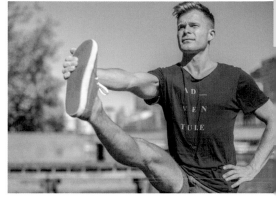

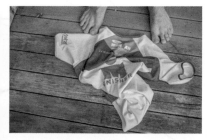

doing. The owner of the studio, who was in the class at the time, eventually came up to me halfway through and said it might be easier if I took my socks off!

I keep coming back because on a physical level yoga always makes me feel better. On a spiritual level yoga is my way of connecting with the unseen – a sacred reminder that there is so much more to this life than what the eye can see and the body can touch.

Tell us about a time your yoga practice came into play off the mat? During an Ironman event I had finished the swimming and cycling components and was starting to lose control of my body during the run – about ten hours into the race. I felt delirious and nauseous, and I was losing control of my bodily functions. The only thing that kept me moving forward was a disciplined concentration on my breath.

What's your favourite pose? Downward-facing Dog. It's my favourite pose to check in because it requires a sensitive balance between strength and softness.

@duncanyoga
Read more at boysofyoga.com @boysofyoga

135

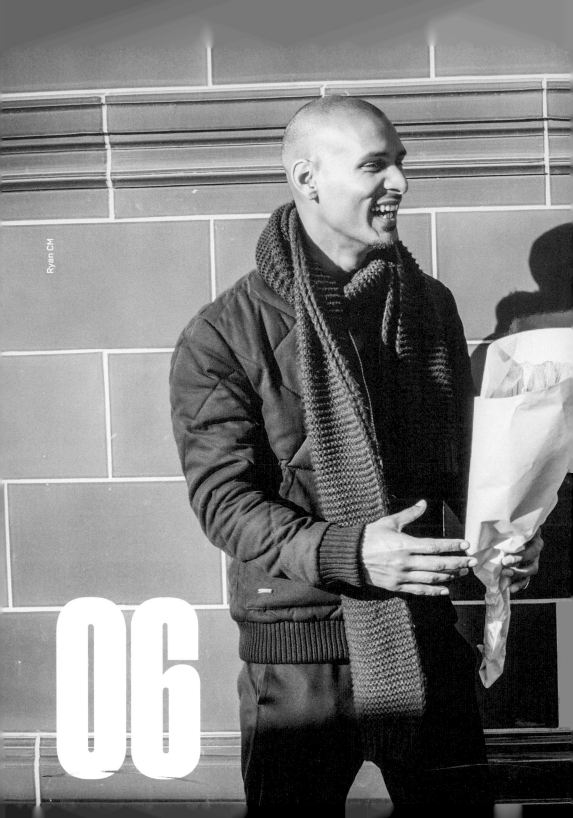

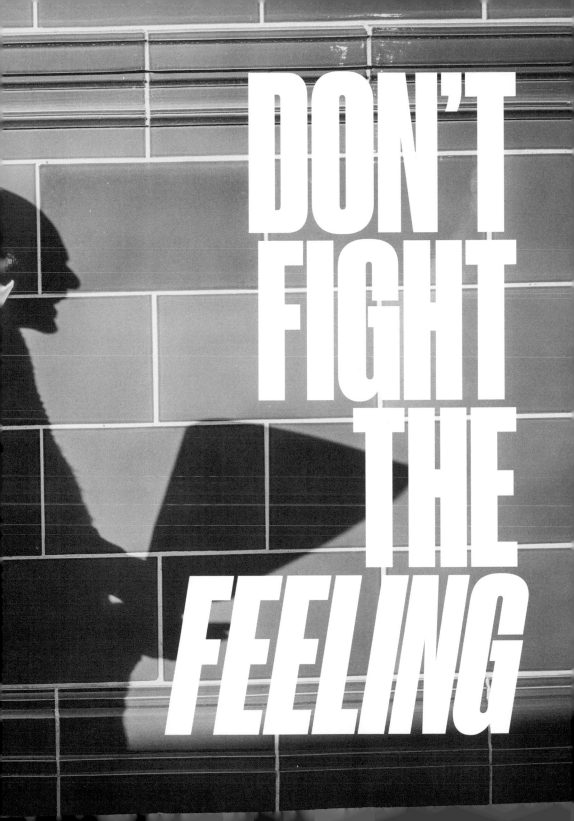

Redefining Manly

For guys, it often feels like there is an unspoken code of conduct to live by – I know I felt this growing up in Los Angeles. Act tough, don't cry, win at everything, show no emotion, don't compromise. This is a common definition in our society of being manly. These characteristics have been passed down from generations before us, each time reaffirming the attitudes and approaches of an out-of-date guide to being a man.

But what if that's not you? Are you less of a man than others? I know I struggled with this growing up. I wasn't the toughest kid, I cried any time things didn't go my way and in reality, I didn't really care all that much if we won or lost during high-school sports games. I was just happy to get on the field and play. As a society we lose sight of the fact that these stereotypes stunt the growth of our children and add the shackles of manly expectations. In effect, we are asking half of the human population to act like 'men' instead of themselves. This is insane.

It's time to wake up. We're now in the 21st century and being a guy isn't what it used to be. And it's great. It's time to redefine what it means to be a man for today's society, for the now.

We live in a progressive world in which we can each make our own choices about how we live and act. We're in a new era where we have the freedom to rethink the old and appreciate the new.

I believe the new definition of a MAN should be simple:

Mindful, **A**ware, **N**on-judgemental.

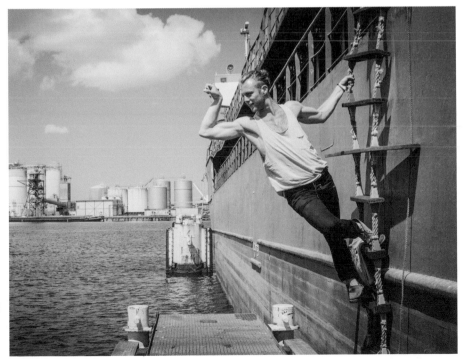

Nicholas Higgins

Crying Is Not A Weakness

At what age did we learn that guys shouldn't cry? Because at some point, as we 'grew up', it was ingrained in us that it's not ok and we learned that showing our emotions like this doesn't have a place in our day-to-day lives.

Often we bottle up our feelings and don't let them out. We sacrifice how we feel because we believe we mustn't show weakness. And that's the biggest misconception. Crying is not a weakness. For me, it's an emotional and physical release that is necessary to both physical and mental wellbeing.

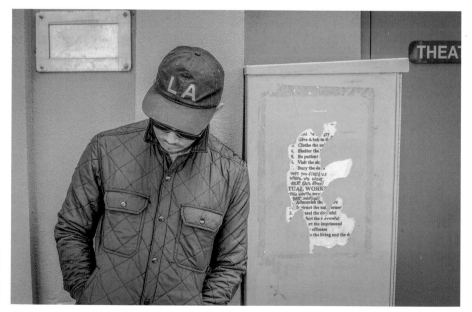

Marco Antonio

Shut Up And Dance

As guys, we all make excuses. Sometimes big ones, sometimes small ones. And sometimes we make them to get out of things that scare us or make us feel awkward . . . Like when we are asked to dance.

I'm talking about real, uninhibited, free-flowing, arms flying, hair-whipping, head-banging, crazy, foolish dancing. The kind you might do at a wedding, fuelled up on liquid courage.

For a lot of us there is something holding us back. Yes, we can feel the beat, we're not robots. But, for some reason, there is always something restraining us.

If you're not that type and you're the first to get your groove on, that's awesome. Keep dancing. The world needs more guys like you.

But for the rest of us, there is a little voice in the back of our heads (our ego) that stops us from getting on the dance floor. So we make excuses. We convince ourselves it's a good time to go to the bar or bathroom, or to take a call. Or we just stand awkwardly on the sidelines, smiling and nodding along. This is the safe zone. The no-fun zone. We're on the sidelines, not living, just existing.

But we're the only ones missing out. Everyone else out there on the floor is having a great time. So if this is you, don't let your ego win. Get out there and dance, enjoy the moment, enjoy your life. The simple truth is, no one actually cares what you do or what you look like when you're dancing, it's all about the feeling that you can enjoy. You should be dancing for yourself, not anyone else. And that's the way it works in yoga, too.

In life, we can always say NO. We don't need a reason or explanation. NO is a full sentence, but YES may be the start of a new adventure. Experience is everything in life. So say YES and see what happens. Do the things that scare you, have fun and don't take life too seriously. It's said that you only have two breaths that are guaranteed in your life: your first and your last. What you do in between is up to you, so why not make the most of every moment and say YES more often.

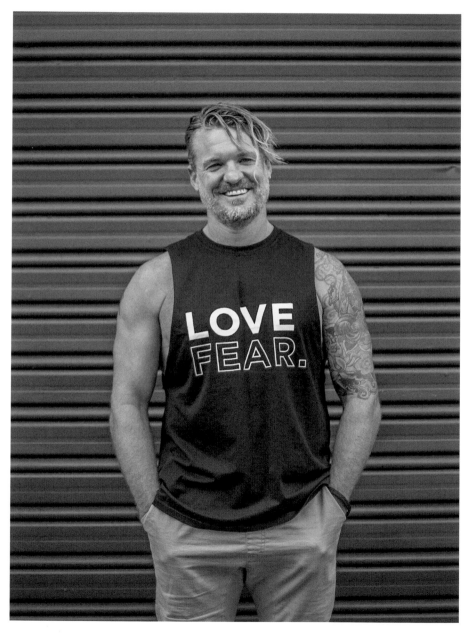

Please, Thank You, I Love You, I'm Sorry

These are the four most powerful statements I can think of, each filled with positive intentions that connect us to each other and show we care.

Sometimes we take these words for granted, though, which can mean that we often take other people for granted, too. But with a mindful outlook we can turn this around and cultivate true appreciation in each other. Gratitude is a feeling, not an action, and one that we should practise daily.

Please and thank you

When you stop and think about it, please and thank you are optional phrases in our dialogue. They're not essential words for communicating with others, so we have to make a conscious choice to use them.

Please represents respect and the acknowledgement that no one owes you anything. It's not just a pleasantry if we understand the reality of its usage. Similarly, thank you recognises your gratitude and appreciation to others – for their time, their services and their attention.

I love you

I love you is a big statement. Many of us save it for special people and special occasions. But why? We save it for our mothers and significant others, but rarely say it to our friends, classmates, students and people we meet for the first time. But why can't we love everyone? Love is not a scarce resource; it's endless, abundant and always readily available. We can give and receive love all day, every day. We shouldn't be limiting our appreciation of others.

Maybe these days the words 'I love you' have loaded connotations. But I believe that 'I love you' simply means 'with the greatest of appreciation'. To love someone is simple. Don't overcomplicate it, and say it regularly.

I'm sorry

When was the last time you said this and actually meant it? When was the last time those two little words came out of your mouth? If you can't remember, you either say it a lot or you don't say it enough.

Humans can be defensive creatures. We don't like to be wrong or have our egos threatened. Saying sorry isn't natural for many people, and apologising can be uncomfortable at times because we must first acknowledge we have done something to offend someone else. So what do we do instead? We argue, offend, offer alternative perspectives, become dismissive or just keep talking for the sake of it. For so many of us, this is easier than saying those two little words. We believe the words 'I'm sorry' admits defeat and can be filled with shame.

But what is wrong with saying that you're wrong?

Saying 'I'm sorry' is owning your words, actions and decisions. It's acknowledging first within yourself and then having the courage to acknowledge it to others. Humility is a powerful quality to incorporate daily.

There is an old saying about facing hard times or a challenging situation: 'It's like paddling upstream without an oar'. Have you heard this before? My father used to say it to me a lot when I was a kid.

And this is how it often works when no one is willing to say 'I'm sorry'. You're battling opposing currents and moving in two different directions, and neither party is willing to budge. Regardless of who is right or wrong, you're not flowing the same way. Disagreements and arguments always end in a stalemate, but acknowledging the times when you are wrong in a humble and egoless way gives everyone the chance to move forward together. Don't let the boat sink, use an OAR to move forward.

Own it

You can't make a change or right a wrong until you accept that it was you who created this situation. 'I' is a powerful word. It stands alone, singularly, and it represents you and only you. Only when you are ready to stand up and own the fact that the argument is something that involves you and your choices will you be ready to start taking action.

So often we try to say 'we', 'they', 'it'. Start using 'I' and own your situation.

Acknowledge it

We are all different people. Something that's not offensive to you may be so for others. What you believe is firm, others may not think is firm enough. What you think is fair, others may think is unfair. This is the cause of many conflicts: the inability to acknowledge someone else's point of view. By acknowledging their perspective, we are saying: I understand that your way may be different to my way.

Resolve it

Resolution comes next, it's the first step forward. This could be as simple as stating that it wasn't your intention to make them feel bad, or you stating that your attitude and ego were misguided. To resolve the situation is to say 'I'd like to stop creating resistance between us'. When resolution is actioned, we move forward.

And that's it. When you say 'I'm sorry', you own it. These two small words said to someone else are your acknowledgement of this with the intention to resolve it and move forward. Saying the words 'I'm sorry' isn't the hardest part; it's owning it and being willing to move forward, even if it may not be the direction in which we were heading initially.

Remember, all these things take practice, it's the work (and yoga) we do on the inside that has so much positive effect on our everyday lives. This is the real power of yoga – sometimes we just do it off the mat.

In practice:
*I'm sorry, I **[OWNING IT]** offended you and didn't ask you what you wanted to do on Friday night **[ACKNOWLEDGING IT]**. It wasn't my intention to take our planned night together for granted. I just wanted to go out to dinner together with my friends that I haven't seen in a while, so I thought we could have one big party. I'd still like this to happen, but I understand that you imagined the night without anyone else around so we could spend quality time together. I can see how this has created contrasting intentions for tonight. What would you prefer? Spending time with you is the priority for me, everything else is a bonus. **[RESOLVE IT]**

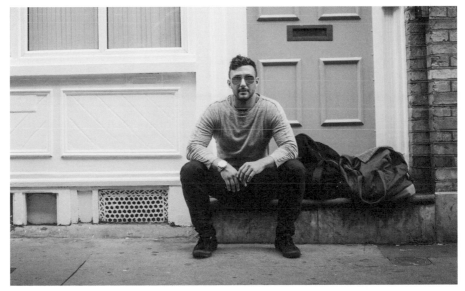

Anwar Gilbert

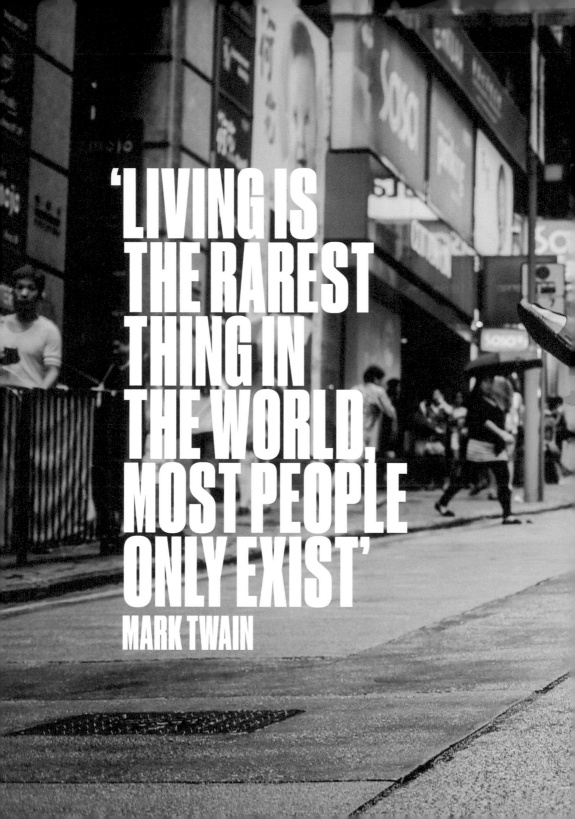

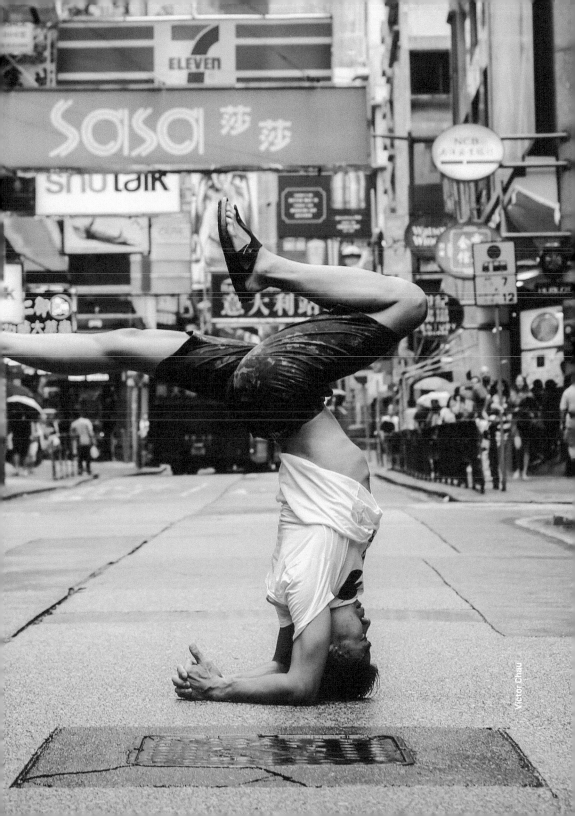

Victor Chau

MEET THE BOYS

ADAM WHITING

NORTH CAROLINA

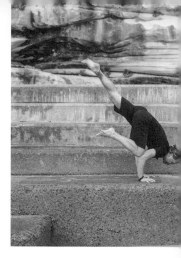

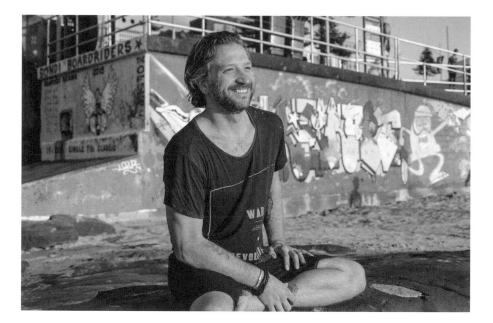

What's your story? I spent my school years in a conservatory studying classical guitar. After seven years of intense study, I blasted off to New York City and started my journey as a musician and, eventually, a yogi. My days were spent working odd jobs and practising yoga. My nights were spent writing, recording and performing my music.

@adamwhitingyoga
Read more at boysofyoga.com
@boysofyoga

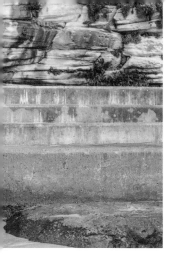

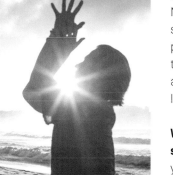

**MUSIC MAN.
COFFEE ADDICT.
INTROVERT.
YOGI.**

How would you describe yourself? It has taken a long time for me to be able to embrace my tendency towards introversion. When I'm not teaching, I lean towards the quieter side. I believe I stepped into my power when I embraced that and stopped trying to fight to be something else.

What do you value most in others? I value integrity. I value people who wake up every morning and strive to be good people – to live simply and honestly. And I value people who expect the very same from me.

How did you get into yoga? When I was living in New York, I was struggling with post-traumatic stress disorder (PTSD), which included battles with panic attacks and depression. I searched for ways to alleviate the symptoms, including medication, and only found a true path to healing when I started practising yoga.

What was the biggest challenge when you first started? I was very aware that my body wasn't yet capable of the fluid, graceful movements that I was seeing around me. I have always been self-conscious about my body, and being a novice in a packed yoga studio only exacerbated that.

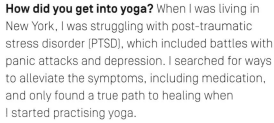

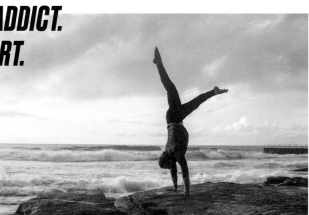

MEET THE BOYS

GISLI GUNNARSSON BACHMANN

ICELAND

What's your story? I was the goon in school, always trying to make sure everyone was happy and having fun. I started athletics when I was ten and then took up karate at 12. I would classify myself as a martial artist that switched to yoga. I had plans to be a doctor, but just before I was about to go to medical school I put them on hold and moved to Thailand for six months to study Muay Thai kick boxing. I postponed my studies even further after that and travelled for the next five years doing whatever I could think of. During this time I got my yoga therapy certificate in India and started teaching.

What characteristic do you value most in others? Vulnerability and humility. The ability and strength in others to be themselves and know themselves.

Why do you keep coming back to yoga? I just don't feel the same without it. After knowing how good it feels when I practise regularly and consistently, I always have that comparison to when I don't. Without it I'm always worse off.

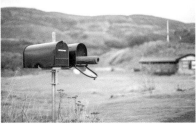

VIKING. GOON. SHAOLIN PHILOSOPHER. YOGI.

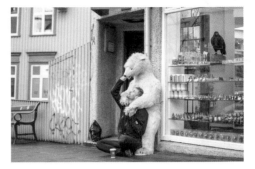

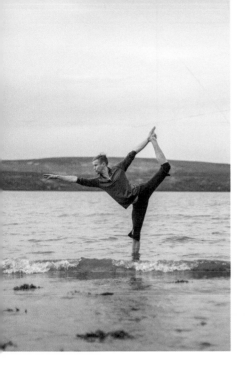

What is your advice for a guy who wants to try yoga for the first time? Give it a real shot and not just one time. Commit to a few classes and do them or else don't bother. You're going to feel terrible the first time because it's going to be awkward, tough and painful, and you'll think everyone will be judging you. But by going a couple more times, you work through your initial insecurities and start feeling the real gift of it.

Tell us a story about when your yoga practice came into play off the mat?
Saying I love you is a big thing in Iceland; it's often so awkward that people won't do it. For example, my mum will sometimes write 'I love you' to me in English simply because it's too much to do so in Icelandic. She really loves me, but it's just so awkward and unnatural. My dad, to my memory at least, never told me straight out that he loved me. I hadn't said it to him either, or at least not for a very long time. Yoga gave me the courage to know better, so I started saying it. At first I was hesitant, but it grew on me and I got better and better – so good that I was able to tell my dad that I loved him. And he finally said it back to me and meant it. I can't tell you how much that meant to me.

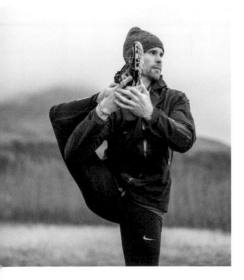

@gisbac
Read more at boysofyoga.com @boysofyoga

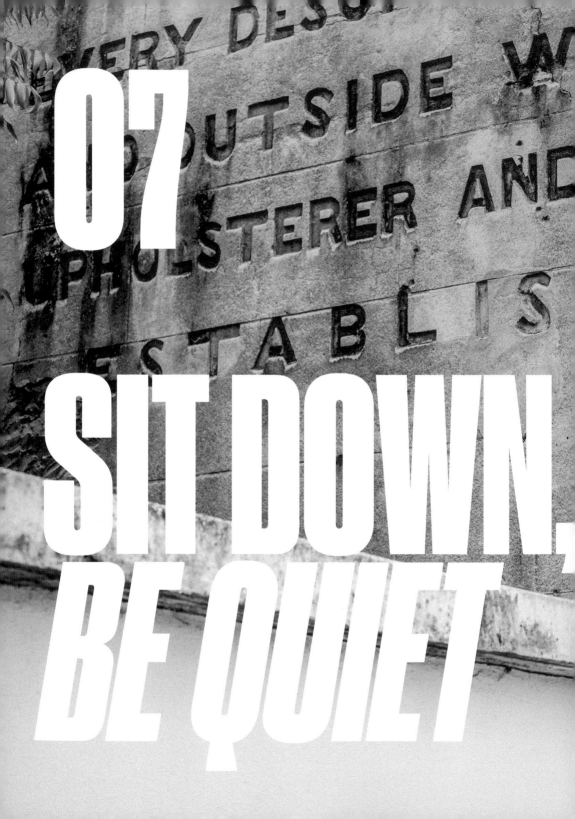

07

SIT DOWN,
BE QUIET

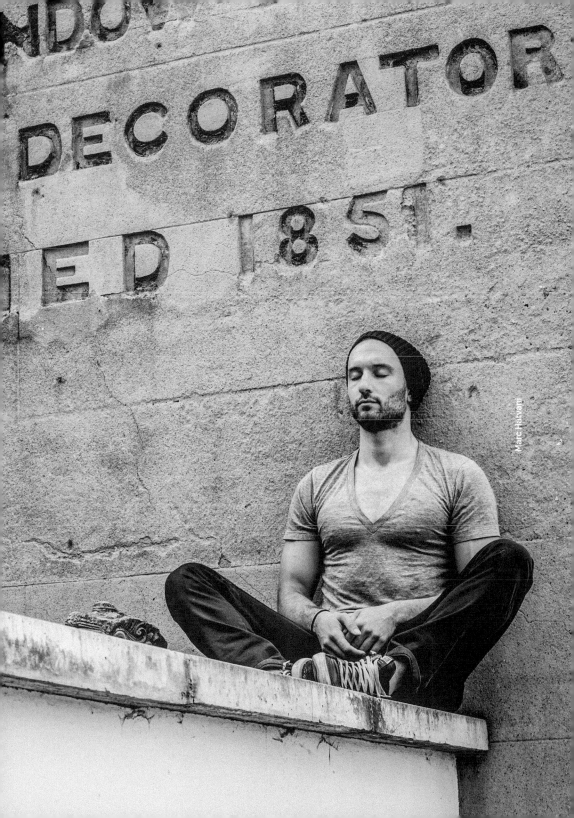

DECORATOR

ED 1851.

Marc Hatvani

Turn The Volume Down

We live in a noisy world where everything around us is always switched on. We are always receiving stimuli in one form or another – noise to the ears, smells to the nose, touch to the skin, colours to the eyes, taste to the tongue. This is how we make sense of the world.

It's easy to get overloaded. We allow so much to come in, rather than blocking some of it out, and sometimes it overwhelms us. This is how stress and burn-out happen.

We need to turn the volume down.

Talk Less, Listen More

The best place to start is to stop. Talking is one of the noisiest things we do. We create noise every time we open our mouth, and we create noise in our head, every time we prepare to speak, and in doing so, we minimise our ability to receive. When we talk we don't listen. The brain works in a way where the moment we have something to say, we stop listening and start getting ready to talk. Cognitively, when we stop talking our ability to hear actually becomes far more acute.

The art of listening is just that. It's an art that we should not take for granted. Did you know, to listen – to really listen – is to stop creating words or formulating a response; it's allowing yourself to be present, alert and attentive to the conversation you're having. Too many of us are already formulating answers and responses in our heads long before it's our turn to talk.

An exercise in active listening

Next time you're in a conversation, focus your attention completely on listening. When the person you're speaking to has finished, simply say, 'Thank you for sharing,' and then pause.

Take a moment to think back to what they said: how it made you feel, the thoughts that came into your mind. Remain quiet for a few seconds and then create your response.

Continue your conversation this way and see what happens.

Yes, it will take longer, but maybe for the first time in a while you'll actually listen and hear what someone else has to say.

Listening is more than what you do with your ears

The idea of 'talk less, listen more' is much bigger than a single one-to-one conversation. Listening is about appreciating the right here, right now.

To listen is to notice and pay attention: to what others say, to how we feel and to what we need. In life, we talk a lot to each other and to ourselves. We're always talking. But how often are we really listening?

Let's change that.

Sit Down, Be Quiet

When was the last time you sat still? Was it intentional? How quiet were you really?

In this chapter we're going to talk about meditation and the practice of finding stillness every single day.

We all know people who do a million things at once. You might even be one of them. They juggle work, social events and side projects, they carry on two conversations at the dinner table and their fingers are always non-stop scrolling on their phone. If they're in a yoga class, they're probably attempting to do everything. But when it comes to sitting still, it's just not for them. In fact, it's almost impossible. It may even annoy them or they may feel that it's a waste of time. Even when they think they are doing it, they're still doing something else; the mind is still thinking and doing. They can't switch off.

For them, sitting still is hell on earth. And I should know – I used to be just like this.

Sitting still is hard when we first start. We can always find something that needs to be dealt with, or something else that needs to be done right now. Carving out a space every day for a moment to pause just never seems high on the priority list. But why can't we prioritise doing nothing? Why is it so hard?

Most people haven't taken the time to try. It's too daunting. But if that's you, what do you have to lose? Sitting quietly is never a waste. Giving yourself time to focus within, instead of being distracted by the outside, will always have a positive effect in your life. By finding stillness you can create a sense of calm in your mind and body. This is the practice of modern mindfulness and meditation. It takes dedication and work to find the time, but it's always worth it when you do.

Start simply. Close your eyes and be still. Let the mind rest. Calm the senses and focus on the inside. Meditation can have immediate effects on the mind and body. Physically, it slows us down and challenges us to do less. Mentally, it allows our mind to actively rest, which we rarely do. Active rest is a conscious choice to put the minds into a state of ease. There is a big difference between meditation and sleep.

There are many types of meditation and some will suit you better than others, but any type is better than none. On the next page you'll find one to get you started.

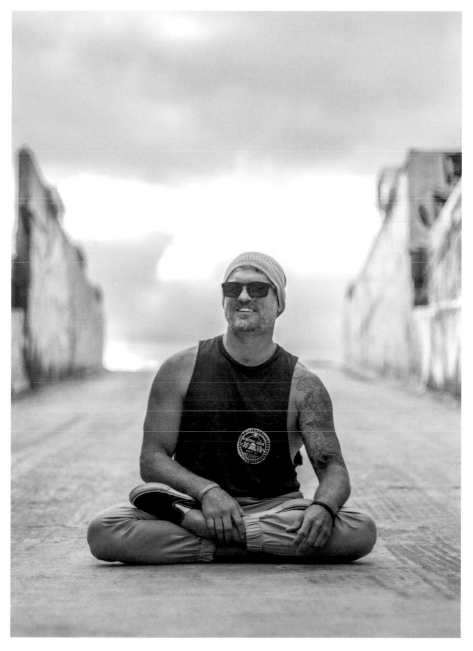

Duncan Peak

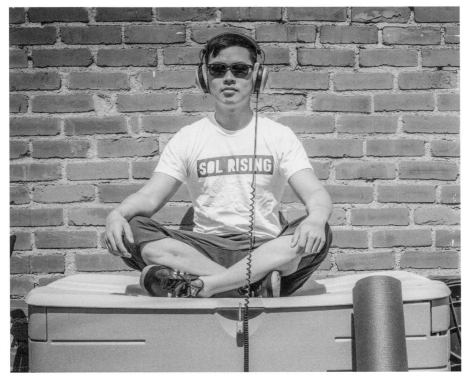

Sol Rising

Real World Meditation

Starting a meditation practice can be daunting. Sitting down, shutting your eyes and doing nothing for 20 minutes can sound like an eternity. And for many of us, when we first start, it feels that way, too. But there is no such thing as a 'good' or 'perfect' meditation.

There are many styles of meditation, some shorter, some longer, but for this practice we are going to aim to sit and breathe for 20 minutes (twice a day).

Why 20? It's often said that 20 minutes is the ideal length of time for the body to rest in calmness to receive the full benefits of the practice. After this you've reached 'rest saturation' and any additional time doesn't offer as much benefit. It's like your phone: once it's charged, it's charged, no matter how long you leave it plugged in. This length of time respects and reflects many of the ancient traditions of meditation practice.

While you may be worried that 20 minutes is quite a long time, when you think about it it's really only 1.4 per cent of your day.

But fear not, if you can't find 20 minutes, then do 11, and if you can't do 11, do 5. And if you can't find that, then you may need to check in with your priorities because it sounds like you really need to start meditating.

Here are some guidelines to get you started:

1. Find a comfortable place to sit, where you won't be disturbed. You don't need to be cross-legged on the floor or change into your yoga clothes; you just need to be somewhere you can be comfortable (a steady armchair or sofa, at your desk, sitting upright in bed or, if you want, sitting easily on the floor or leaning against the wall). It's also nice to remove your shoes.

The best way to sit is any way that is comfortable for you, where your physical posture is not distracting.

2. Set a timer. This is a great way to hand over control, so you don't have any reason or excuse to cut your time short. Make sure you pick an alarm that is gentle. A sharp exit from a meditation is like getting a bucket of ice-cold water dumped on your head in the middle of the night.

There are many good meditation apps with timers that will give you a gentle notification when the allotted time has passed, so do yourself a favour and download one to your phone. JUST BREATHE is my recommendation, which you can find easily in the app store for free on most smartphones.

Add 20 minutes to the timer and get ready to sit. During the first stages of the meditation your body will adjust and settle, so allow yourself a few breaths to calm the body and find ease in your seat.

Here's an analogy to explain this. Imagine your friend offers you a cup of tea, and you accept. They bring it into the room and put it on the table in front of you. The cup is still, but the tea inside is still moving around. It takes a few moments for the tea to settle and the ripples to subside so you probably don't start drinking it straight away. This is similar to how the mind works. When we first sit to meditate, the mind needs a moment to find stillness.

3. Minimise the external distraction where possible. While it's not imperative that the room is completely silent, it's helpful if there is nothing obviously distracting. Leave your baby with your partner or other adult, move away from loud music, turn off the television. Giving yourself the best chance for stillness by removing these external annoyances will serve you well. But don't worry if there are things you can't change or turn down. Just do what you can. Anything is better than nothing.

20 MINUTES
TWICE A DAY
JUST BREATHE

4. Close your eyes. This is the hardest part for a lot of people. Actively closing your eyes for the duration of a meditation will seem impossible when you first start. Your mind will flick into overdrive and you'll wrestle with every fleeting moment until it's over. But trust that the time will pass faster and faster every time you practise. Closing your eyes is just one more way to avoid distractions.

5. Breathe and let go. It's time to begin. Bring your attention to the breath, slow and steady with a gentle and natural inhale and exhale. This is all you need to do.

At times the mind will wander and you may find yourself lost in thought. But

the aim of any meditation is to let the mind be at ease, so while we focus on the breath, we don't force control. If it helps, you can recite to yourself 'just' on the inhales and 'breathe' on the exhales. This may help you to keep your focus narrow and mind clear.

At the end of your meditation, don't spend any time analysing what happened; just simply appreciate how you feel now your eyes are open. If you feel refreshed, calm, energised and light, then the meditation was good, and therein lies the benefit.

And if you don't, know that it wasn't bad. It was just an experience that didn't serve you well today. The best thing, regardless of how you feel, is to do it again tomorrow.

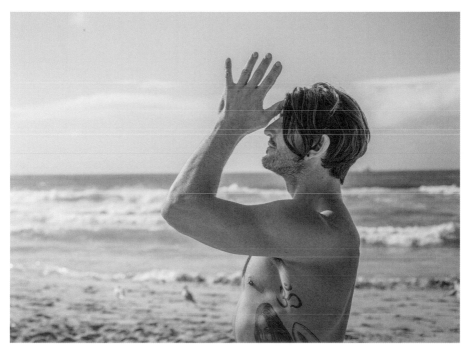

Johnny Vasilj

Cultivate A Quiet Conversation

As you create time to sit still and meditate, you'll see how stepping away from the noise is truly beneficial. Cultivating quiet as a lifestyle approach will affect everything you do. Your edges will soften, your expectations will ease and your desperation to fill space with your words will dissipate. These days, I notice a big difference in how I act and am. I enjoy long moments of no talking, I don't have anxiety about small talk; I can just enjoy the silence. Once you step into stillness, you'll wonder how you ever operated in such a noisy world without reprieve.

MEET THE BOYS

JONNI POLLARD

MELBOURNE

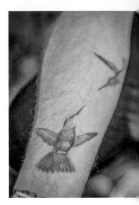

What is your story? I'm a simple guy with a deep sense of purpose to awaken the full potential of what it means to be a human. I travel the world sharing the knowledge I've gained from great masters about how to become embodied. I take great pleasure in all things creative, elegant and expressive of our higher nature. I'm fascinated by the process of human awakening and see the last 22 years of studying and teaching as the foundation for at least another 60-years-plus of discovering new frontiers of our humanness.

How would you describe yourself? Surrendered, accepting, inclusive, loving, present, insightful, capable, silly.

What do you most value in others? I value people's sincere heartfelt present attention more than anything. This is the only place we ever get to meet each other and connect with the fullness of our hearts and make meaning of our humanity.

MEDITATOR. ICE-CREAM LOVER. MAN IN THE MIRROR. YOGI.

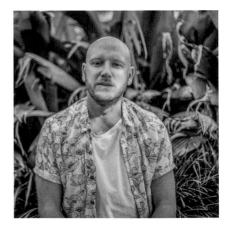

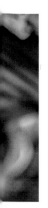

What advice would you give to someone stepping onto the mat for the first time?
Have fun, let go of expectations, enjoy the ride and after each session sit and meditate for 20 minutes. The whole point of asana is to prepare the mind and body to transcend who we think we are and experience what we are – unbounded awareness with the unending propensity to love and be compassionate in the face of fear and defensiveness. We are immeasurably powerful and the practice can reveal this power very quickly.

What pose do you hate and why? The poses I pull in the mirror when I'm trying on something new, trying to create an image of what I think I should look like.

My practice is to stand in front of the mirror and smile at myself. It's very effective in establishing a deep connection with myself as the world might see me. Even if you have to fake it, do it! It will reveal where your heart is at in an instant. Connect with that, good or bad, and be that in front of the mirror. It's powerful stuff, fellas.

@jonnipollard
Read more at boysofyoga.com
@boysofyoga

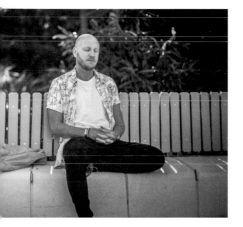

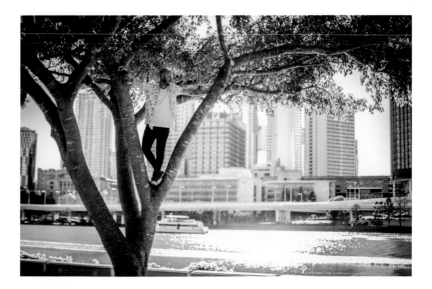

MEET THE BOYS

JONAH BROWER LYON

NEW YORK

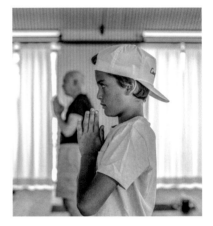

What's your story? The first time I was in a yoga studio I was six weeks old, so at this stage of my life I've been around yoga for about 11 years. I was born in NYC – it's my home, but I've got homies all over the world.

My mom, Elena Brower, is a yoga teacher, so I've been lucky to hang with some great people in cool places. My favourite place to hang with the yoga crew is at Wanderlust festivals, and Australia is pretty bomb.com.

I'm an athlete – I play hockey, soccer, baseball, (American) football, basketball and my favourite team is the New York Rangers.

I'm a DJ. I go by DJ Pulse. My beats are electronic and rap. I'm pretty sick.

I'm also a classical pianist. I've been playing for seven years, and I practise for one to two hours every day.

What does yoga mean to you? To me, it's the different environments, the teachers and all the nice people I get to hang with.

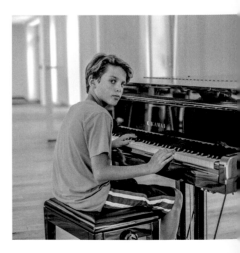

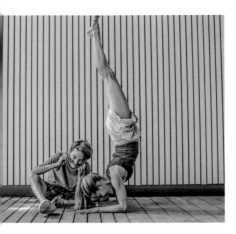

HOCKEY GOALIE.
PIANO PRODIGY.
NEW YORKIN'.
YOGI.

What is your best advice for a dude who wants to try yoga for the first time? Never be pressured to do yoga, just have fun and be chill. Wait for the right time and take your friends with you, but don't go to your mum's classes.

Tell us a story when your yoga practice came into play off the mat? I think that yoga will change the world because it teaches us to be nicer and to treat other people with respect.

What is your favourite quote, or personal mantra? 'When plan A doesn't work, you still have 25 more letters in the alphabet, so take a chill pill.' – Jonah Lyon, not Yogananda

Why do you want to share your story? Because I want to be a part of the BOY project and let kids my age know that yoga is cool.

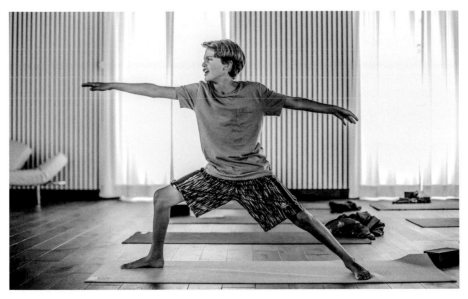

@jonahlyon
Read more at boysofyoga.com @boysofyoga

MEET THE BOYS
DANIEL SCOTT
SAN FRANCISCO

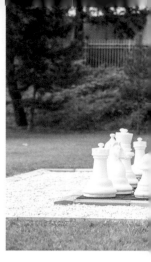

MOUSTACHE MAN. WHISKEY CONNOISSEUR. YOGI. ALL OF THE ABOVE.

What's your story? Anything is possible at any time, given the right combination of effort, desire and resource. Let's just say my favourite answer for multiple-choice questions is 'All Of The Above'. I was voted 'Most Unique' in high school ... which was a HUGE compliment, considering I grew up in a particularly homogenous, middle-class suburb in the Tri-State area. Competitive swimmer, professional lifeguard and Vice President of the video yearbook in High School; model student by day, party promoter by night – a mix that continued well into my years as a young professional afterwards.

What was the biggest challenge when you started practising yoga? Finding a yoga teacher who 'spoke my language' (less frou-frou, more Let's Do This). Hilariously enough, all I could find were guys who fit that stereotype (natch) or women ... who also fit the same stereotype. It took a lot of trial and error to find a teacher who spoke directly to my sensibilities and interests. A LOT.

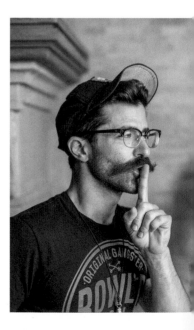

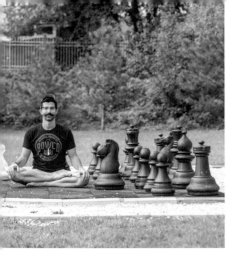

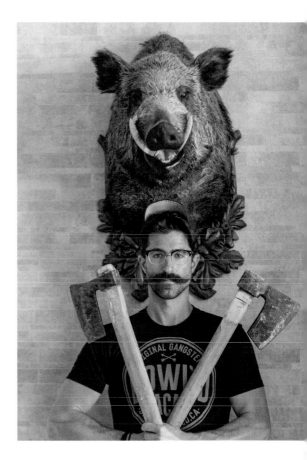

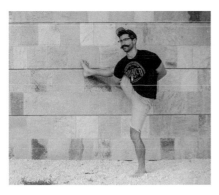

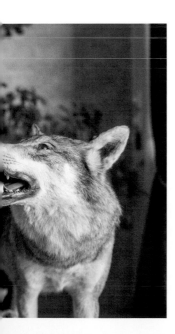

What is your best advice for a guy who wants to try yoga for the first time? Don't worry about how it looks, bring awareness to how it feels. All those other people in the room? They don't really know much more than you do and nobody knows your body better than you.

Tell us about a time when your yoga practice came into play off the mat? Most recently, I had to deal with the DMV (Department of Motor Vehicles) and nobody got hurt. Plus one for YOGA!

@danielscottyoga
Read more at boysofyoga.com @boysofyoga

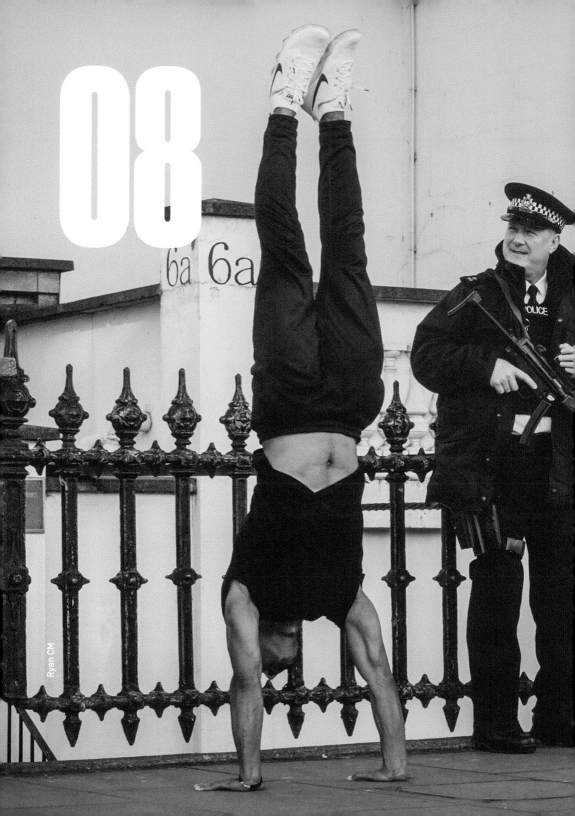

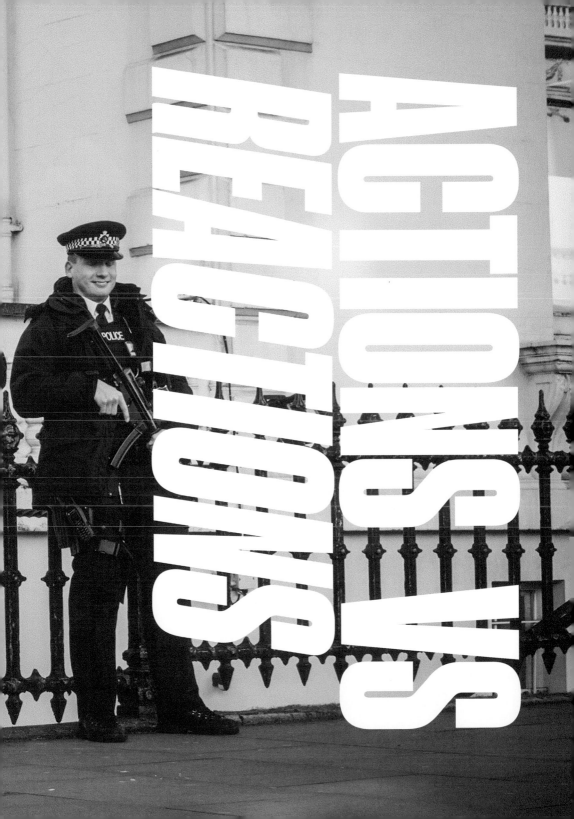

ACTIONS VS REACTIONS

What Is An Action?

Webster's Dictionary defines it as 'a thing done'. I like this definition – so simple, clear and concise.

An action has two distinct phases: an intention and execution. Before we act, we must first have intention: 'What is our purpose for doing this? What are we hoping to achieve? What is the motivation behind it?' Only then should we execute: 'What is the best method for getting it done?'

This process applies from the smallest of actions to the grandest, and can happen hundreds of times every day, often in a split second.

Say you're hungry. You don't just magically get full – you must first eat something. This is an action: you act by eating some food. But before you do that you have a clear intention.

Let's break it down.

The problem: I'm hungry

What is the intention? If I eat this sandwich, I won't be hungry.

What is the execution? Make a sandwich, eat the sandwich and now I'm not hungry.

Do you recognise the stages? They may happen almost simultaneously, but each stage is there. With clear intention, our choices in execution are considered. Oftentimes, without the intention we simply react without thinking and the outcomes can be less than ideal.

So what is a reaction? A reaction is a response. It's an action that usually affects us and plays on our tempers

'CHOOSE WISELY, LIVE WITHOUT REGRETS AND LEARN FROM EVERY EXPERIENCE'

and egos. Put simply, a reaction is a regrettable action. It is something we do with impulse or instinct and at times often regret later. Reacting does not allow us to make the best choices in the situation; we just make a responsive choice.

Does this sound familiar? How many times have you said something reactively, something you probably didn't mean but it ended up coming out anyway?

How many times did you regret it?

In yoga, on the mat, we move carefully, consciously and mindfully placing our bodies into postures and positions with full awareness and accountability, and in life we should be doing the same.

No Regrets

The idea of regret is one we all know and try to avoid. Regret isn't a good feeling because we know we could have done better or achieved a more positive outcome.

We're human. We don't need to be perfect, but we can do our best to see how our choices and actions best serve and support our lives, instead of regretting those we made when reacting to something. There are some things in life that you can't take back, so action carefully.

But what is regret?

For me, regret is the idea that we should have done something differently. It's often quite clear after the fact that our choices at the time could have been different. Sometimes it may have been our egos getting in the way, or choices we made in the heat of the moment – these are the moments that we define as regret.

But what if we defined our actions differently? Rather than labelling them as regrets, what if we acknowledged them simply as experiences to learn from? Yes, we can all acknowledge that our choices could have been better, but regret keeps us looking back instead of moving us forward. With a simple shift in approach, we can start to live life without the burden of regret.

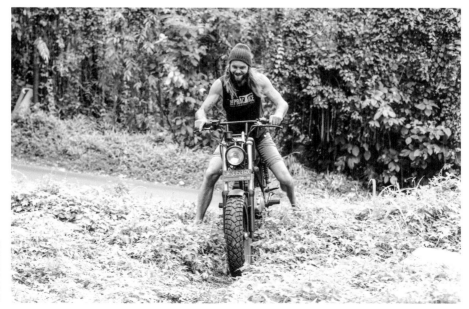

Octavio Salvado

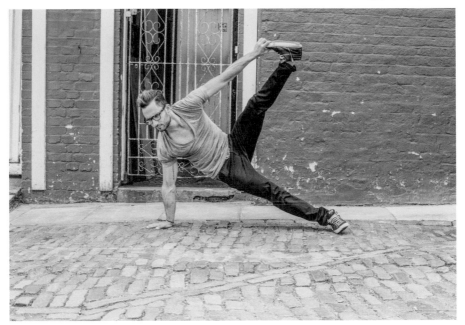

Marc Hatvani

How does this apply to yoga?

In yoga we always move consciously, manoeuvring our bodies into postures and positions with awareness and accountability. But there will be a time where you might go too far, or push too hard. Often this results in injury that may sideline your practice for a day, or weeks. This has happened to me plenty of times over the years and to many yogis I know.

Once, I fell while I was in Crow pose. I wasn't paying attention, my hands slipped and I twisted my wrist. I couldn't practise that pose for almost six months. It would have been easy to get angry, regret the decisions I made when I was practising, try to blame the teachers for giving me the option to try something different or just let the frustration win. But the truth is, these were my actions, my choices and my decision, regardless of how mindful I was in my actions. I may not have liked what happened, but looking back, I learned something about myself. The experience wasn't pleasant, but it was valuable.

I now know my limits, and I now always approach this pose with my full attention because I know what will happen if I'm not aware and mindful of my actions.

So choose wisely, live without regrets and learn from every experience. This is how we can live mindfully every single day.

MEET THE BOYS
TRAVIS ELIOT
LOS ANGELES

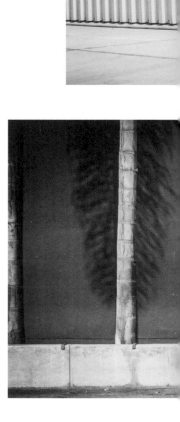

What's your story? I was born in Texas and grew up in North Carolina, where I started meditating at the age of nine. I worked in the entertainment business for a while before discovering yoga, then, after a near-death experience in Kauai, Hawaii, things really started to shift for me and I began to dive deep into all things yoga.

What's the biggest challenge or issue being a guy who teaches/practises yoga? In LA lots of guys practise yoga so it's become pretty normal, which is so awesome to see. But sometimes when I travel for a workshop it's almost all-female and, although I have no problem being around a bunch of ladies, I can see how guys get put off by that. They think it's just for the girls! I understand because I had the same initial resistance. But once you can get past that stereotype, you can see that yoga is open and beneficial to everyone; a lot of my friends/students are professional athletes and they all do yoga. I think the key is to find the right teacher and the right vibe of a class for you.

Yoga is... freedom. Every human being is looking for freedom. Some do it through negative means and others do it through positive means. But we all want to be free. And yoga helps us achieve this.

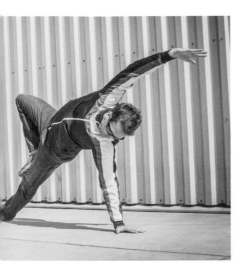

BEACH BOY.
MANTRA MAN.
MUSICIAN.
YOGI.

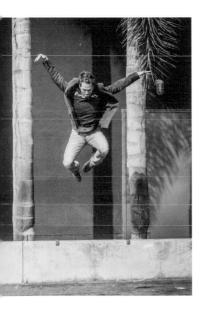

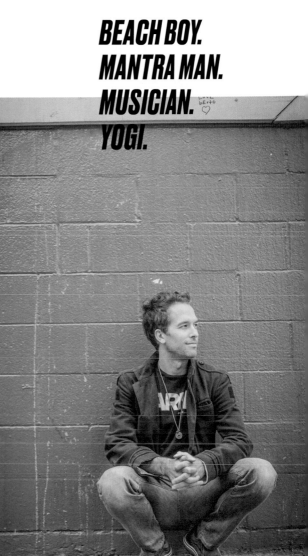

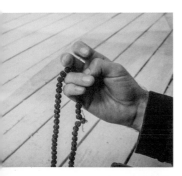

@realtraviseliot
Read more at boysofyoga.com @boysofyoga

MEET THE BOYS

OMAR SULTANI

DUBAI

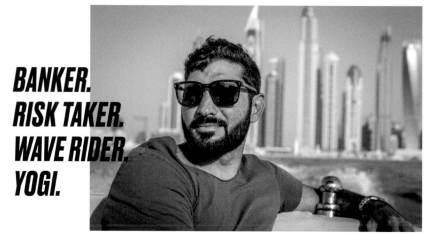

BANKER.
RISK TAKER.
WAVE RIDER.
YOGI.

What's your story? I was born in Libya and moved to Beirut as a kid, but due to political instability in both countries my dad moved us to the UK. I spent my childhood and teenage years in London. I graduated from an American School and went to college in Boston. My first job was working as an analyst for a bank. After that I moved to Japan and was a teacher for a few years, then moved back to the West Coast and settled in Portland, Oregon, before relocating back to the Middle East, to Dubai. I love travelling and learning new things. I'm a perpetual student of life.

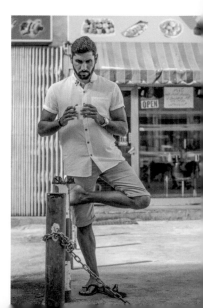

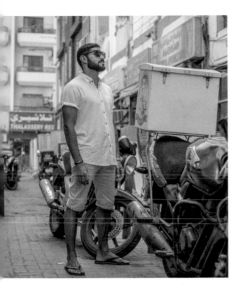

What was the biggest challenge when you started teaching? Candidly, it was finding the time. Working full time in finance made it initially difficult to commit to a regular class. The thing is, the time is there, you just have to commit to it. I'm so glad I did as it has really made a huge difference to my quality of life.

We've all done a few things we're not proud of. Care to share one? When I look back at the volumes of things that I'm not proud of, they all share one thing – when I've not been true to myself. When I've done something that didn't hold true to my genuine self. Stories that you hold onto from your childhood that made you believe you're a terrible person really aren't as dramatic or as serious as you think.

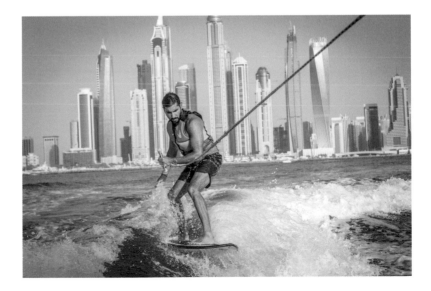

@omieslice
Read more at boysofyoga.com @boysofyoga

MEET THE BOYS

CHARLIE KELLY

LONDON

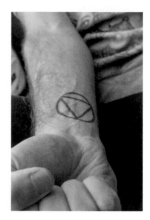

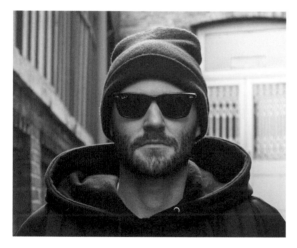

RAVER.
TRUTH SEEKER.
TOOTHBRUSH HATER.
YOGI.

What's your story? I'm a born-and-bred Londoner but went to nine different schools (some boarding schools) growing up. I came back to London fully when I was 15 to pursue mind expansion, but at that time the only way I knew how was through chemicals (some natural and others not so much). I was involved in the underground dance and psyche-trance scene. Eventually (as you might expect), it got out of hand and I decided life would be better if I gave up drinking and using.

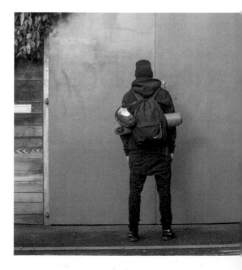

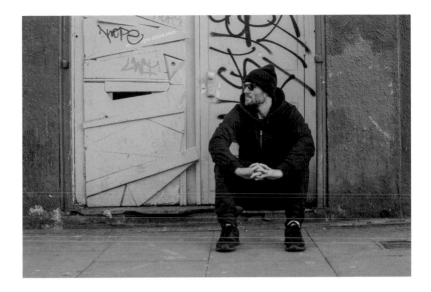

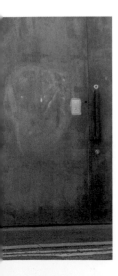

Read more at boysofyoga.com
@boysofyoga

What's it like being a guy who practises and teaches yoga? I love the practice and I love teaching. I love telling people who are new to my class that I can't touch my toes, and then watching the worry lift from their faces, especially the guys. Yoga just rocks. It's a place where I can come and sit, stand, twist, bend (kind of) and breathe into my life situations. There is also a wicked, beautiful, loving and inspiring community that I just love being involved with.

If you could do it all again, what would you change? I would not have cared as much at school. I allowed the social pressure to achieve to weigh too heavily on me.

What is your personal mantra? 'Om gam ganapataye namaha.' This bad boy removes any obstacles in life, in the mind and spirit – anything standing between you and a higher and more connected experience.

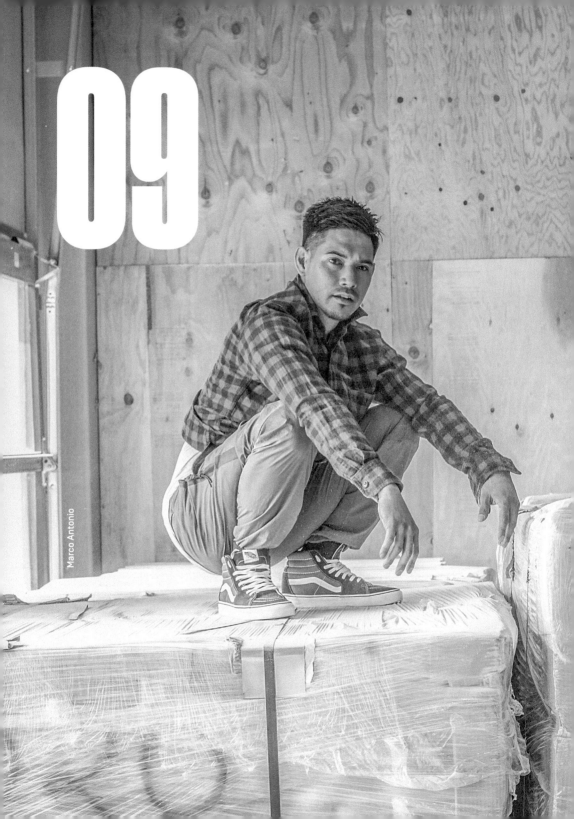

09

Marco Antonio

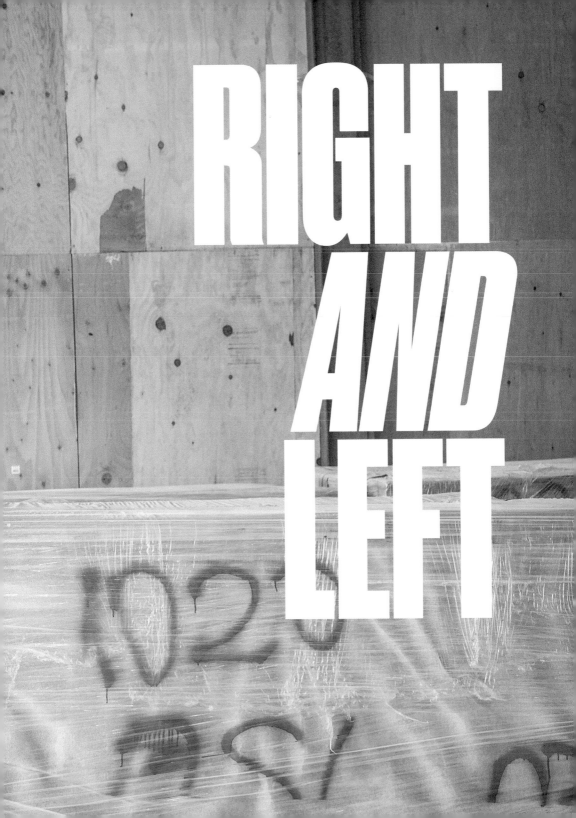

Not Right And Wrong

'Life isn't about right and wrong – it's about right and left.'

The first time I heard this, it blew my mind.

I was in a yoga class practising with a friend [Marc Laws, one of the BOYS] and he shared this idea. I had never heard it before, but it was a game changer for me. It has changed how I receive everything in the world today.

As humans, we have a tendency to see things in black and white: there are things that are 'right' and things that are 'wrong'. We're not born this way – we learn from a young age. We must acknowledge that this is not a natural thing – it's something society ingrains in us.

As far as I know from my research, around 90 per cent of all people are right-handed. And since this is the majority, most things in our everyday lives are structured this way. We have right-handed door knobs and phones that swipe right and countless other things intentionally built for what's 'right'. But does right always mean correct?

And what's so wrong about a left-handed guitar?

As a society, we have created a definitive system of learning that is rooted in negativity. We have things that are right, and anything else is wrong. But when you stop and consider this thought, we can likely agree that it doesn't always work that way. Our system is broken and we don't even realise it.

Left is not wrong; it's just different. And while it may not suit the masses, it shouldn't be discounted or seen negatively. Others may not always agree with the status quo and instead choose to go left, and that is ok.

Embracing this idea can change everything. You'll find more kindness and compassion will come into your everyday life, and – the best part – you'll find more of these qualities in yourself.

Acknowledging that we all have different opinions, thoughts and perspective is how we understand that nothing in this world is definitive. We all live our lives in a way that works for us, with morals and beliefs we believe in.

That's the practice of yoga in our lives every single day.

Finding The Balance

We're all in search of balance: in our bodies, our jobs, our relationships and with our time. We're always looking for it but we never really find it. We're overworked, over-stimulated and underappreciated, and we can't seem to get off the treadmill. The belief that you don't need to rest is worrying; the ability to bring more balance to life is essential for our wellbeing.

Life is about adjusting to change

Balance is not a destination to arrive at. Balance is not about standing still in perfect stillness; it's about adjusting to change as it comes. Balance is doing what is necessary to find calm, compassion and happiness in the moment, even in chaos. When you start trying to cultivate balance in your life, you'll find that it's not always easy.

Think about when you first learned how to drive a car. You gripped the wheel tight as you tried to keep the car on track. But every time there was a tiny movement or bump in the road, it felt like the whole earth was moving beneath you. Dealing with the change was draining. You may have only gone a mile down the road before you were physically and mentally exhausted. You were holding on like crazy thinking you could control everything, and you probably weren't breathing.

This is not balance. This is trying to control the chaos.

Now, think about when you're in a yoga class. The teacher announces Tree pose – to the uninitiated this looks calm and elegant. Well, often, it ain't like that. In fact, it feels like at any moment the tree is going to fall down or worse, snap in half. It's more like the 'stand on one foot, cramp in your calf, wobbling like a giraffe at the ice rink, sweating or crying (you're not sure) wondering how long are we going to be here', kind of pose.

The truth is, to find balance you must always keep adjusting to find the least resistance. The aim of balance should always be to move with ease and adjust to the change as it comes (like the wind through the leaves of your Tree pose).

This is balance in the real world.

Albert Mordue

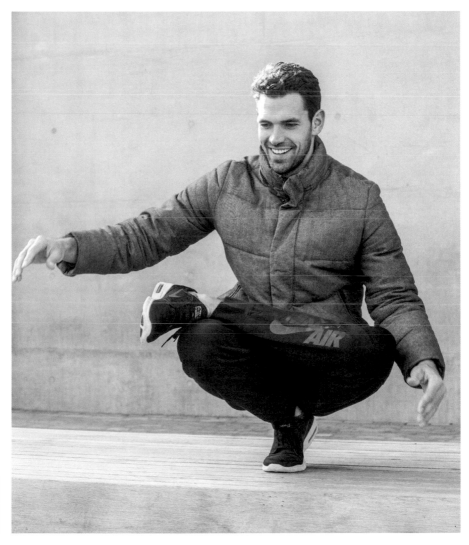

MEET THE BOYS
MATT GIORDANO
CONNECTICUT

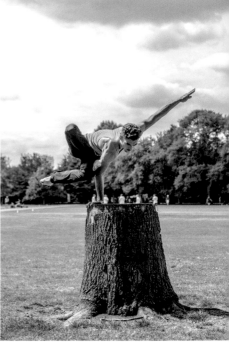

What's your story? As a kid I wanted to be an actor, but reading was never my strength. Reading out loud for auditions was so embarrassing that I avoided the whole process. Stage fright was also a limiting factor. Still, I knew self-expression was important to me and in my late high-school years I fell in love with music and art. I went on to study music at college and toured nationally in a band called 'Stealing Jane' for eight years. We had some success, but the challenges of working as a team with a total of eight dudes, lacking in maturity, life experience and communication skills all while making big life decisions eventually caused us to fall apart. We did our best and learned a lot together, but the unsteadiness (to say the least) of that lifestyle led me into depression. Throughout my final years in the band I started a meditation and self-inquiry practice which eventually led me to a book, *Wisdom of The Peaceful Warrior*, which, in turn, led me to yoga.

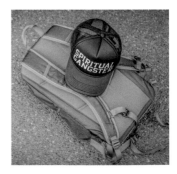

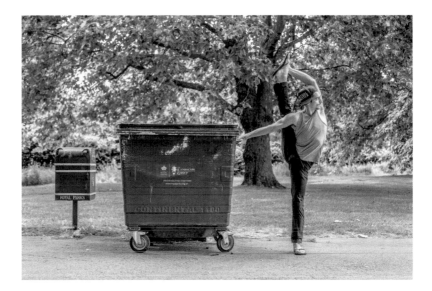

REBEL ROCKSTAR.
KOMBUCHA DRINKER.
PEACEFUL WARRIOR.
YOGI.

@theyogimatt
Read more at boysofyoga.com
@boysofyoga

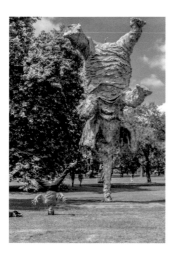

We've all done a few things we're not proud of. Care to share one? Just one? I was fired from a big clothing company for stealing ... but that wasn't the only time it happened. I went through a rebellious phase where I stole just to see if I could – money, posters, clothes, CDs and so on. To say I am not proud is an understatement.

What is your best advice for a guy who wants to try yoga for the first time? Most guys face their own inner critic, self-doubt and judgement when thinking about going to a class for the first time. My advice is to muster up the courage by focusing on how you want to feel rather than what you think you will look like. Like anything, you can't just be good at it without working at it. You won't be flexible after one practice, so keep at it.

MEET THE BOYS

MARC LAWS II

LONDON

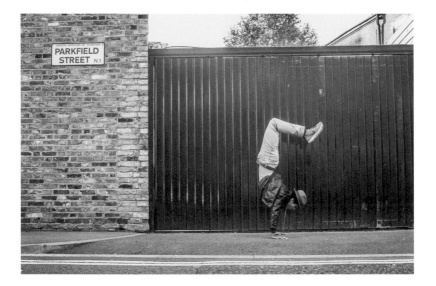

What's your story? I was born in England to a Canadian mother and an American father. I have African, Native American and Ukrainian roots, and think of myself as a citizen of the world. From England we moved to Ottawa, then to California and finally landed in the beautiful and enchanted land of Albuquerque, New Mexico ... I grew up playing football, and my dream was to play in England. I'm thankful that I was able to fulfil that dream in my early 20s.

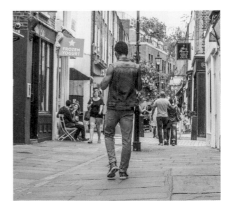

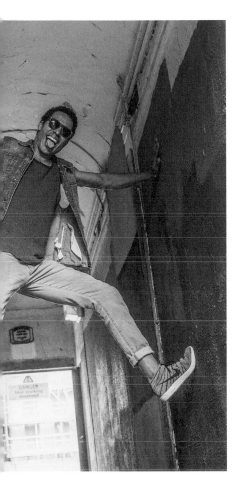

What's the best and worst job you've ever had?
My mum wanted me to learn a lesson about the value of money and the power of education, so she made me get a landscaping job. I wanted to be on the creative side of landscaping, not the digging-of-trenches side, but that wasn't really an option at the time. On that job I met and worked with loads of immigrants. These guys were badass and super hard-working; my work ethic didn't compare. On top of that, these guys were sending their money back home to feed their families while sharing a room with four or five other guys.

It opened my eyes to the things I was taking for granted, and I developed a strong sense of disagreement with the invisible lines that mark all these territories we call countries, since they only create separation. I came to understand love expressed through sacrifice. It was one of the hardest jobs I have ever had, but I was taught some of the greatest lessons I've ever learned.

What was the biggest challenge about yoga when you first started out? Not pushing myself too hard too fast.

What is your personal mantra? Never look down on a person unless you're helping them up.

PRO FOOTBALLER.
STARGAZER.
LOVE MAKER.
YOGI.

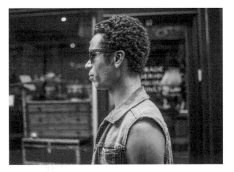

@marclawsii
Read more at boysofyoga.com @boysofyoga

MEET THE BOYS
DUSTIN BROWN
MELBOURNE

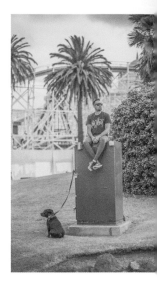

What's your story? I grew up on Kauai, Hawaii (heaven on earth), surfing every day and living the surfer lifestyle. I then moved to California in my 20s. After a few years, the stars aligned and I packed my bags and started travelling the world and surfing professionally. I met my wife, Nova, in Melbourne, Australia, which quickly became home. Winters were cold, so I soon needed a new sport other than surfing to keep me active. A Hawaiian friend introduced me to Brazilian jiu-jitsu and I was instantly hooked. My love for yoga came a few years later – my body was sore from Brazilian jiu-jitsu and my wife convinced me to go to a class with her. I loved it and felt it complemented my surfing and grappling. My wife and I opened our own yoga studio in Melbourne in 2015 and I am now expressing my passions through teaching jiu-jitsu and yoga every single day. Life's good.

Favourite book? *The Power of Now* by Eckhart Tolle. This book changed my perspective on life in a very positive way.

What was the biggest challenge when you first started yoga? Learning to respect where my body was physically and changing my mentality. I went from pushing my body and competing with other people to listening to my body's feedback and working with that.

PRO SURFER.
BJJ ROLLER.
NINJA MASTER.
YOGI.

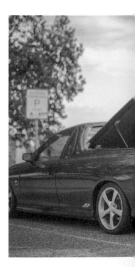

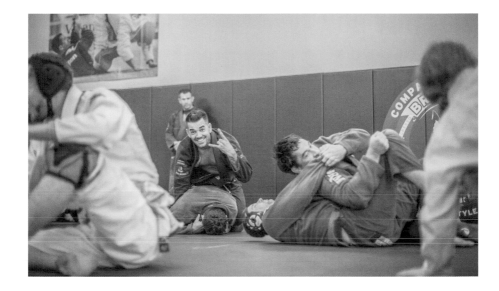

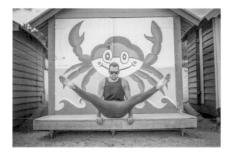

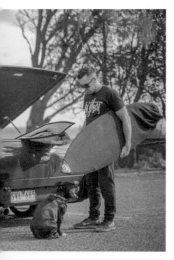

Why do you keep coming back? Every time I show up on the mat my mind and body thank me. Yoga has completely changed my perspective on life, as well as my relationships with others and myself. It's neverending and always evolving, allowing me to give back to myself. When you come from a place of self-love and self-acceptance, only then can you truly give your best to others.

Other than yoga, what keeps you busy? I'm a Brazilian jiu-jitsu black belt so I train every day and teach my team of students in the evenings.

What advice would you give to someone stepping onto the mat for the first time? Yoga is a journey of the self. There is no competition with others. You don't need to be anything but you. The goal of yoga isn't to control your thoughts; it's to stop letting them control you.

@dbrownyoga
Read more at boysofyoga.com
@boysofyoga

MEET THE BOYS

JASON ANDERSON

ATLANTA

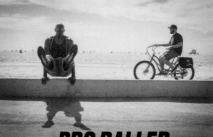

PRO BALLER.
VEGAN.
HUMBLE WARRIOR.
YOGI.

What's your story? Professional basketball player turned professional yogi.

How would you describe yourself? Tall, dark and handsome. Ha ha! Seriously, though, I'm a gentle and quiet soul within a strong physical build. A loyal friend to those who are loyal friends to me. Focused. Talented. Moody. Both secure and insecure. A fast learner. Courageous and fearful. Creative. A lover and a fighter. Graceful. Composed. A loner, but not lonely. Disciplined. Vegan. I like to hug. A teacher and a student. Adventurous. Accomplished. Observant. Imperfect. Protector.

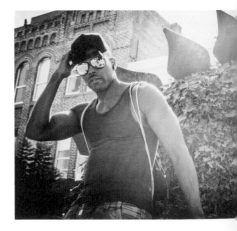

What's the worst job you ever had? I worked at a constructions site one summer. My mother actually made me. I would rather have worked on my game full time. The site was a huge open field of red clay and it was crazy hot and the labour was brutal. It definitely encouraged me to pursue my dreams and not settle for things.

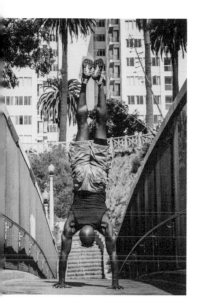

Most embarrassing yoga moment? I was in a very intense power yoga class in a small, crowded room. Hot, too. Remember, I'm like 6ft 6in tall. During a standing forward fold the instructor gave the option of tripod headstand. I saw others going upside down and decided to do it too, without having practised it before. Long story short, I fell out of the pose on top of three people – and someone's glasses. Luckily, nothing but my ego was seriously damaged!

What's the biggest challenge in being a guy who practises yoga? Being taken seriously – as opposed to being seen as some object that just wants to get with all the girls!

@calmtivity2
Read more at boysofyoga.com @boysofyoga

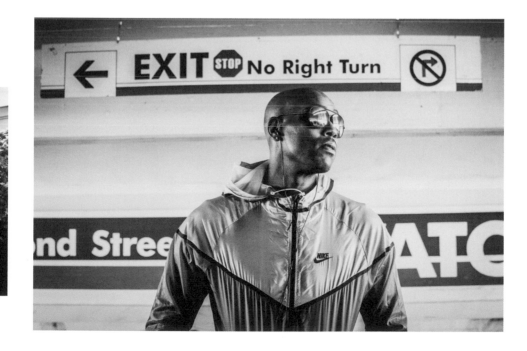

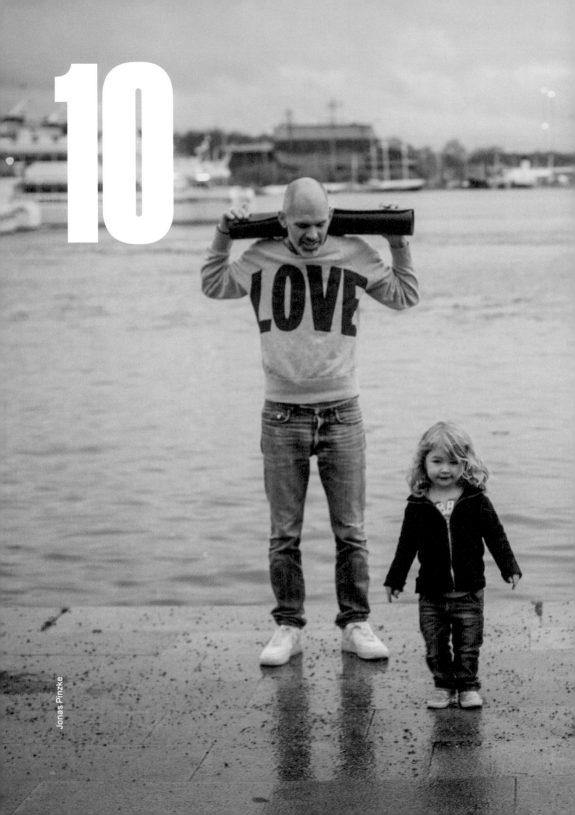

10

Jonas Pinzke

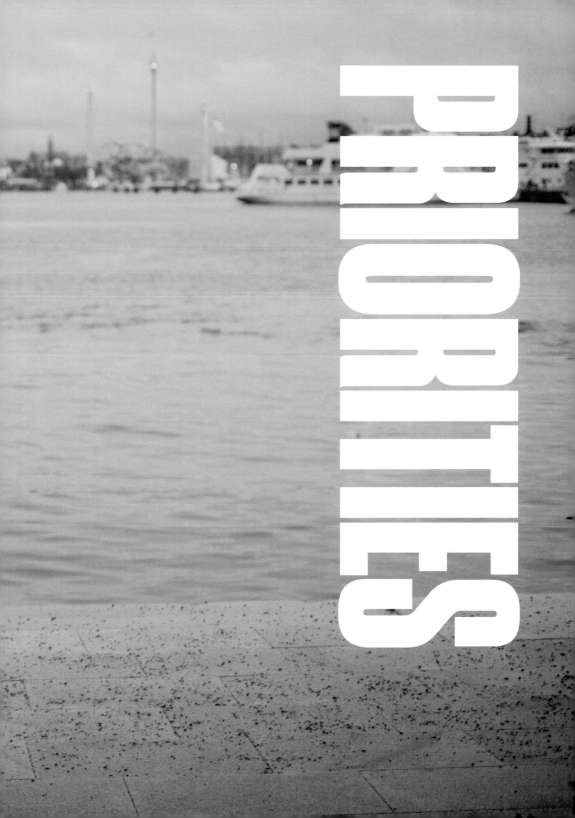

Get Them Straight

'I never have enough time in the day. There is always too much to do.'

How often do we hear ourselves saying this? How often do we feel this way?

When you combine work, friends, family, social occasions, yoga, fitness and general life admin, it can all seem too much and we can easily feel overwhelmed. We're busy people living in a chaotic world. It's a normal human reaction to feel this way: we pile on too much and then spend most of our lives worrying about how to get it all done.

The unfortunate reality is that we usually do it to ourselves, and we do it willingly. We say yes to far too much. And we allow ourselves to get busy.

The real question is: do we have our priorities straight? Or are we doing so much that we don't even know why we're doing it?

Priorities: what are yours?

Stop and take a moment to think about the priorities in your life. Literally stop and write a list. Grab a piece of paper and a pen. Try to be as specific as possible.

What's on your list?

Is it things like:
'Spend more time with my family.'
'Show up for my niece's school play.'
'Go on an adventure holiday.'
'Do the things that make me happy.'

Or is it things like:
'Impress my boss and stay late at the office.'
'Attend every party I'm invited to so I'm in with the cool crowd.'
'Go to my next-door neighbour's barbecue.'

The point here isn't to judge, it's simply to consider and ask yourself the questions that matter.

If your family is more important to you than your job, don't sacrifice story time for office time. If your relationship is more important than your friends, don't skip date night for mates' night. If your education is more important than your social life, don't go to the party – stay in and keep studying.

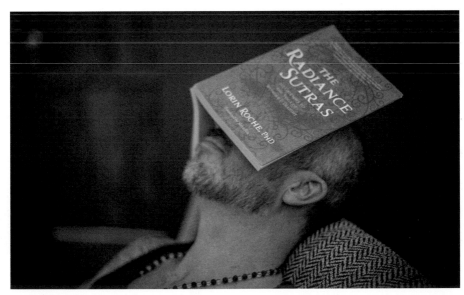

Scott Schwenk

Busy Is A Choice

Think about the last time you ran into a friend you don't see that regularly. It's likely the conversation went something like this.

'Hey, how are you?'

'I'm good. Pretty busy at the moment, but that's life, right?'

Wait, what?

In today's society, busy is a badge of honour – or worse, a marker of success. If you're not busy, you're doing something wrong. But being busy isn't mandatory. It's a choice we make, and taking a moment to acknowledge this is the first step to becoming less busy in your life. When we burden ourselves with so much, it can be tough to figure out how to do less.

The ego has a lot to do with being busy. We allow ourselves to get busy under the guise of ambition. We may believe that we have no choice in the matter. We have jobs, responsibilities and commitments – things we can't change. But the truth is still the same: being busy is a choice. You choose to have that job, you choose to take on those responsibilities, you choose to commit.

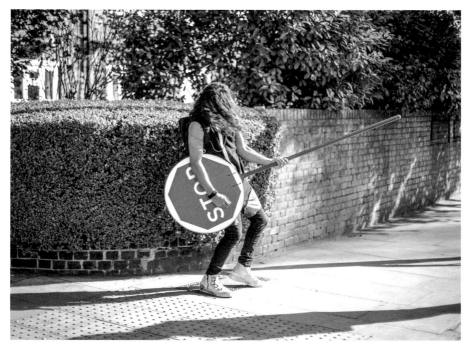

Arli Liberman

Don't blame your busyness on someone or something else. If you're busy, it's because you made a choice to be. Remember, you can stop at any time.

When we look at the concept of being busy, we can see that there are two different and distinct parts: the item and the expectation.

The item is the 'what' – the physical stuff

What do you need to do? What is the action that is required? Do you need to go to the grocery store? Do you need to pay your rent? Do you need to speak to your mother about the upcoming family get together?

The expectation is the 'what will happen' – the emotional stuff

What will happen if I don't do what I need to do? What will happen if I don't take any action? Will I have any food if I don't go to the grocery store? Will I get kicked out of my house if I don't pay my rent today? Will my mother be really upset if I don't call her today?

When we get busy, we often crowd our minds with too much of the emotional stuff, becoming distracted and fearful of the expectations. The fear of 'what will happen?' or 'what will others think?' seems more important than what simply needs to be done right now. If it needs to be done, do it. If it doesn't, don't. And if the expectation of the action is greater than the need for it to be done, then it probably doesn't really need to be done at all.

Understand this and it will be your greatest tool to stop you being so busy in your everyday life.

It's not about having enough time; it's about prioritising the things that are actually worth it. Do the things that matter, the things that need to be done, and don't do anything extra. You don't need to go to the party if you don't want to; you don't need to stay late at the office just to get a head start on the next day. Why take on more when you just want to do less?

Why would you do things that get in the way of your priorities?

Learn how to say no, so that your yes means something.

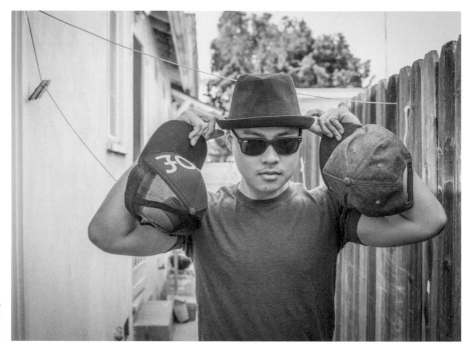

Sol Rising

Do One Thing At A Time, Not Everything At Once

When we are busy, we often can't see through the mess we've created for ourselves. We believe that everything is important and that it will all fall apart if we don't get these things done. Logic is no longer relevant and we're now in crisis-management mode. We've all been here, and it's not a great place to be.

When we get to this point, we're in a state of panic and we exhaust ourselves trying to do everything at once. Or we dabble in our 'to-do' list and spend a lot of time talking about what needs to be done instead of just getting on and doing it.

But when I find myself in this situation, I find the best way to get going is to stop. This might sound insane to you, but it will help. When we stop and breathe we are not giving up or slowing down; we are simply stopping for a moment to assess the best way forward.

KILL THE CHAOS,
MAKE A PLAN

1. STOP AND BREATHE

Slow yourself down and really take a moment to just breathe.

2. ASSESS THE SITUATION

How much stuff actually needs to be done?

3. WRITE IT DOWN

Writing a list lets you see the tasks ahead. Maybe it's not as much as you think – or maybe it's more.

4. REPRIORITISE

Do things in order of importance, not just what comes to mind first.

5. DO ONE THING AT A TIME

Keep it simple. You can only really do one thing at a time, so take the time to do what's needed, complete it and then move on. Too many open-ended things will continue to create chaos.

6. NOW, NEXT, NO THANKS

Use these questions next time you find yourself in crisis mode:
What do I need to do now?
What do I need to do next?
Which things can I
say 'no thanks' to?

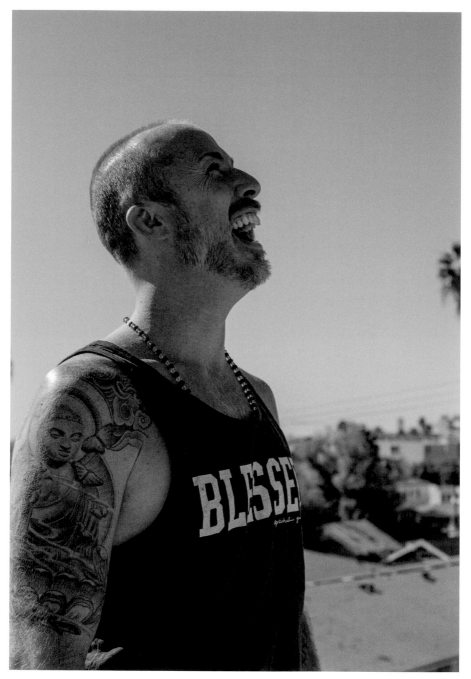

Do What Makes You Happy

This is a story I was told when I was younger, and one that still makes a whole lot of sense today.

There once was a Hawaiian fisherman who lived out on the islands. When he was a young boy his father took him out on the boat to learn how to fish. They were a simple family with one boat, one fishing pole, one net. On that very first fishing trip he caught a fish, a big fish, big enough to feed his whole family. He was beyond happy. When they arrived back home, the whole family sat around for hours laughing, and eating and enjoying the catch of the day. Our young fisherman was inspired and asked if he could go again the next day.

And so the next morning he went fishing again, and again he caught another fish. It seemed he had a knack for it, and each day thereafter he would catch more and more. For the next few years he continued to go fishing with his father and continued to bring back many fish. On most days he would catch so many that he would give some away to his neighbours, sharing the wealth of what they collected from the sea, and in return they would give him a few pennies for his kindness. Soon

he had saved enough pennies to buy a boat of his own, and he believed that with another boat they could double the amount of fish they caught in a day and start selling them at the markets and make a decent wage. His father agreed and soon enough they had two boats and twice the catch.

Over the years our young hero became known as the best fisherman on the island and more and more people would come to the market to buy something from his daily catch. Two boats turned into ten boats, and ten boats turned into 20 and eventually he was the leader of the most successful fishing fleet in all the islands. He had become very successful, very rich and very wealthy.

After some time, the mainland started calling. They too wanted his fish, and they wanted plenty. So, what did our young fisherman do? He purchased more boats, hired more fisherman and sold tonnes of fish to the mainland. Eventually he stopped fishing completely and moved to the mainland to better run the large operation. He was no longer a fisherman – he was now a businessman and his business was thriving.

During the growth of his fleet, he had married and had children of his own, but with such growth and success he couldn't spend much time with his family, and would sometimes go weeks without seeing them. But this was his sacrifice; this was the burden of his

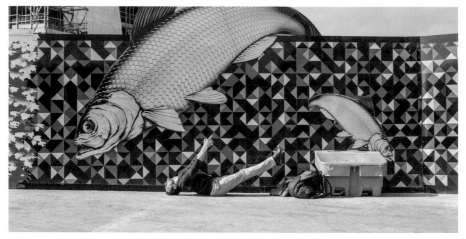

Albert Mordue

business, and this is how he lived for many years.

Eventually he decided it was time to sell the business, and he had so much wealth he now had the freedom to do whatever he wanted.

At the final farewell of his business, his friends and colleagues asked him, 'What will you do now that you can do anything? Will you start a new company, buy a new house, build a new dream?'

The young fisherman, now older in his years, simply said, 'I would like to go fishing'. Everyone was shocked.

'But why? Why would you want to go fishing again?'

His reply was simple. 'It makes me happy.'

And so he and his family moved back to the island that he grew up on, to the same small village, to the same small beach hut. And that very next day he went out on a small boat with his son and they went fishing.

And from that day on, and every day until his last sunset, he went fishing, catching just enough to feed the family, and each night when they got back home they would spend hours together laughing, eating and enjoying the catch of the day.

The moral of the story is this: why do we make ourselves so busy when the things that we love, the passions that we have, are often right in front of us? Why are we always searching for more? If you're already doing the things that you enjoy, with the people that you love, why do you need to do more?

Why do you need to make life busier, when you're already happy with less? Why do we waste the best years of our life remembering the sunrise and chasing the sunset, but never enjoying the moment?

Prioritise your happiness, do what makes you happy and stop being busy.

The choice is yours.

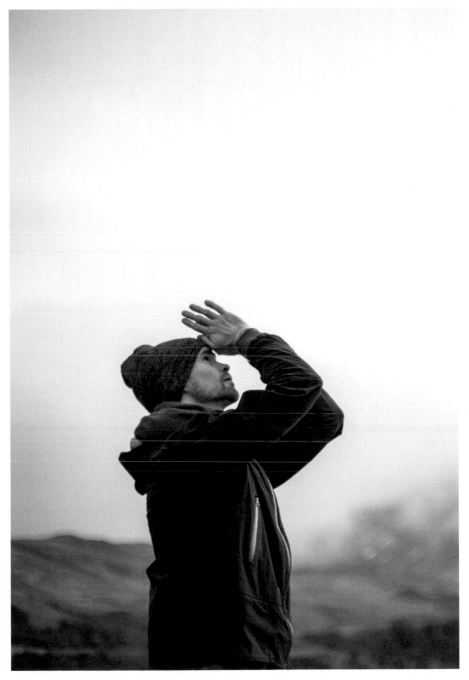

Gisli Gunnarsson Bachmann

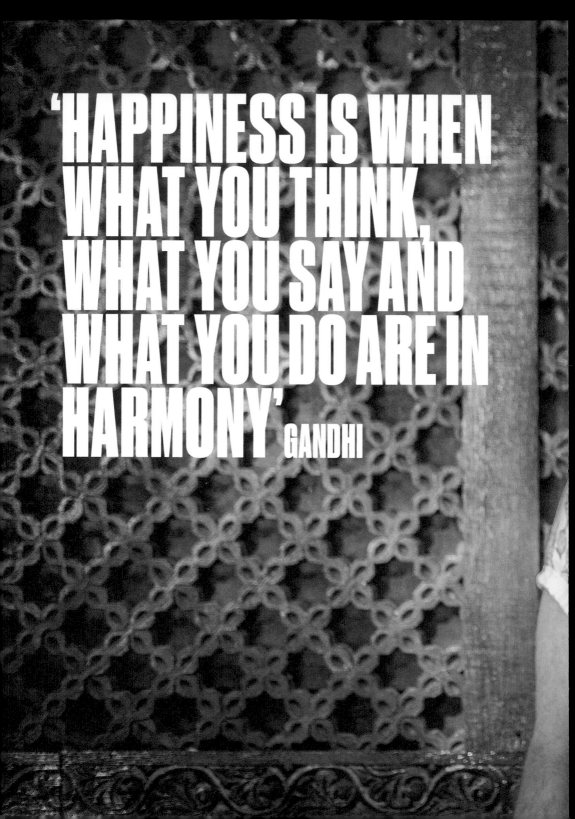

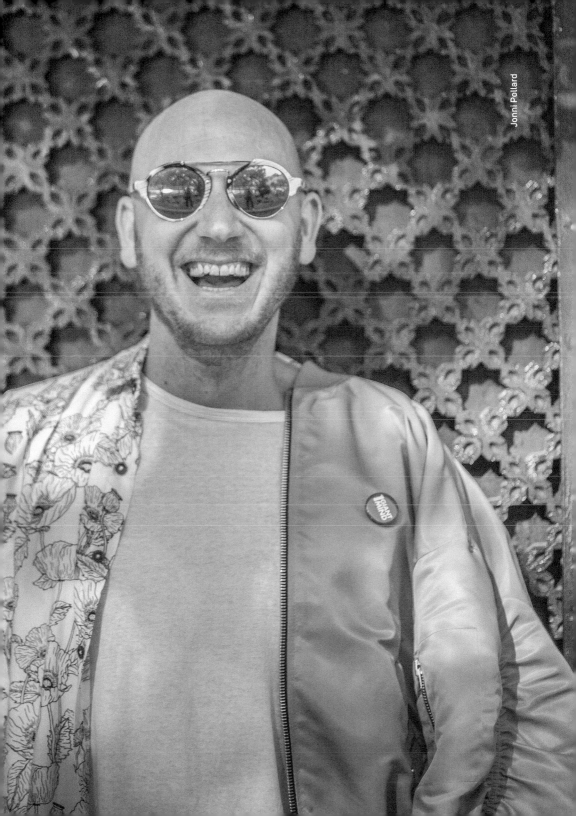

MEET THE BOYS
BENNY GOULD
SYDNEY

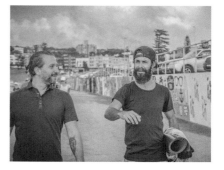

What's your story? Born and raised in the hills of the Dandenong Ranges in Melbourne, Australia, I grew up riding mountain bikes and playing football at the weekend. I wasn't much of an academic, so I decided to leave high school at the age of 17. When I was old enough to sneak into nightclubs and pool halls, I started DJing at house parties and then playing gigs at venues across the east coast of Australia.

People tell me from time to time that I am lucky. This is rubbish. You create your own luck; you just have to be prepared to make the right decisions, no matter how hard that can be.

When did you last cry? Cry? Never ... I've never cried during a lame rom-com at all. Ok, I'm a sensitive guy – let's leave it at that!

What was the biggest challenge when you first started yoga? Judgement. I was so critical of myself. How I looked practising yoga and how I felt in my own skin; feeling disappointed with my own ability. I'm such a competitive person and it is only recently that I learned to let go.

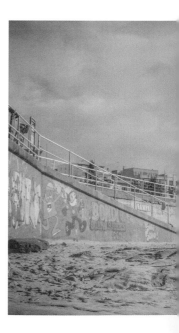

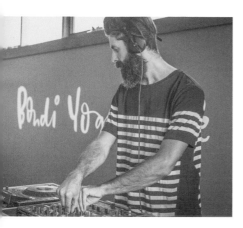

**R&B DJ.
CORPORATE
RUNAWAY.
AUSSIE
BACKPACKER.
YOGI.**

What advice would you give to someone stepping onto the mat for the first time? Live in the moment. No judgement, no expectations. Use the opportunity to learn more about who you are – physically, mentally and spiritually.

Tell us about a time your yoga practice came into play off the mat? I recently met someone in person whom I'd previously known only by reputation and photographs, and, I'll admit, I had them down as a certain type. And it wasn't positive! When we met I realised I'd made assumptions about them that were completely wrong. For me, that was a reminder to let go of expectations and never judge someone or something until you have experience first hand – that's yoga.

Which pose do you really hate? Standing splits and most deep hip openers. I have a lack of rotation in my hip joints and find myself constantly ignoring it and pushing myself. I'm often cursing on the inside, and sometimes on the outside, during these poses.

@bennyjgould
Read more at boysofyoga.com @boysofyoga

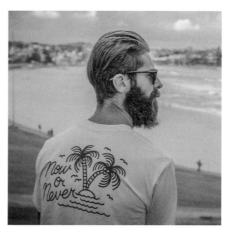

MEET THE BOYS

JONAH KEST

CALIFORNIA

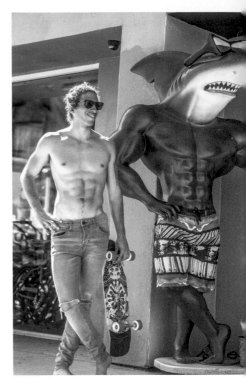

What's your story? I grew up in a yoga family. My dad owned and ran one of the first yoga studios and teacher-training programmes in the Midwest. Ever since I was little, we would always do a gratitude and meditation circle with my brothers before bed. As I got older, I really started to see the importance of a daily meditation and practice. My father was a great example. I started training with him to be an Ashtanga teacher when I was 17 years old. After a few years of studying and training, I began to teach as much as I could and share the practice with whoever would listen. I eventually went to the University of Colorado and taught classes there twice a week alongside my studies. After my first year of school I dropped out and decided to move to LA to teach for my uncle Bryan Kest at his donation based studio in Santa Monica. Yoga is really all I know and I am just grateful it found me. I'm honoured to be continuing the lineage.

How would your mother describe you?
A pain in the ass.

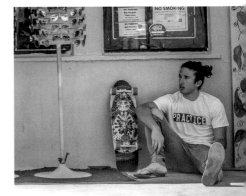

@kestyoga

Read more at boysofyoga.com

@boysofyoga

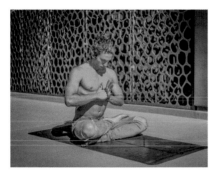

NATURE LOVER. KNOWLEDGE SEEKER. SPIRITUAL GANGSTER. YOGI.

How'd you get into yoga? I didn't find yoga, yoga found me. I was born into it. My dad and uncle are yoga teachers. After years of rebellion, I eventually found a passion for it.

Tell us about a time when your yoga practice came into play off the mat? Yoga has come off the mat for me the most in my relationships. It has taught me to be present, sensitive, make needed adjustments and also not to run away from rigidity but rather soften. These qualities allow you to be in a relationship and come out successful.

What challenges or issues have you experienced being a guy who teaches/practises yoga? Growing up I actually used to be embarrassed because my dad taught my class yoga all the way through elementary school. I thought yoga was for girls. But being a guy who practises yoga has allowed me to actually embrace and strengthen my feminine qualities. This has made me softer, gentler and more sensitive.

MEET THE BOYS

KYLE GRAY
GLASGOW

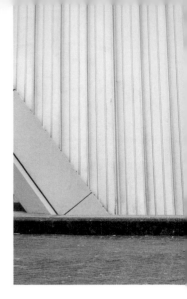

What's your story? I come from a very spiritual background. I had lots of psychic experiences as a child and was encouraged to follow an intuitive path. I was paralysed as a kid – a virus left me in a wheelchair and I had to learn to walk again. Around the same time, my grandmother was battling cancer. I was close to her and this experience left me wide open, sensitive and extremely emotionally aware.

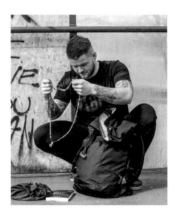

For a long time, I felt like I didn't fit in, like I was an outcast in the world because of my spiritual side – the psychic moments and this intense sensitivity to everything. I had a strong inner practice – meditation and awareness of spiritual principles – but I wasn't united; my soul and mind were getting stronger but my body was extremely overweight. My biggest interest is angels – not in the sense of fluffy winged beings, but more the personification of universal energy.

How would you describe yourself? I'm a bit of a rebel, outspoken and fiery – but I'm all love!

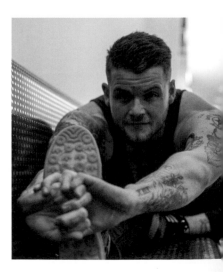

What do you most value in others? Integrity. It's key for me. Speak your truth.

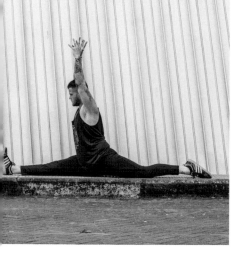

We've all done a few things we aren't too proud of. Care to share one? I recently lost my temper at a parking attendant who gave me a ticket while I was helping an 80-year-old lady into her car. My ego felt bruised that he could do that while I was being of service. I swore lots and lost my mind for a moment. I got into trouble for it, but, more significantly, it was a real lesson for me to stop being so self-important. I've since written an apology letter.

How did you get into yoga? I was overweight and wanted something that would help me get back into shape while honouring the spiritual connection.

ANGEL GUY. BOOK SCRIBBLER. CHEEKY B*STARD. YOGI.

Do you teach? I wanna do it for the larger lads. So many people are overweight and don't go to yoga because of it. They think it's only for the super-lean and strong, but yoga is for everyone. I still have a little belly and lots of stretch marks and I'm proud to go shirtless and show these notches that I have acquired on my journey.

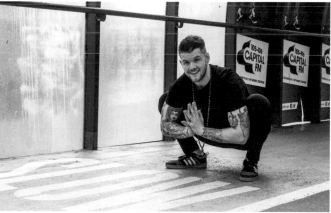

@kylegrayuk
Read more at boysofyoga.com
@boysofyoga

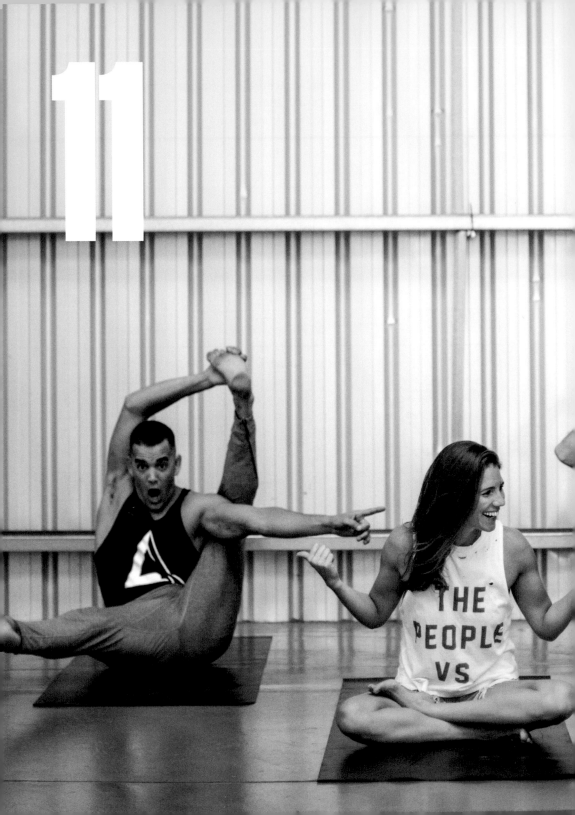

11

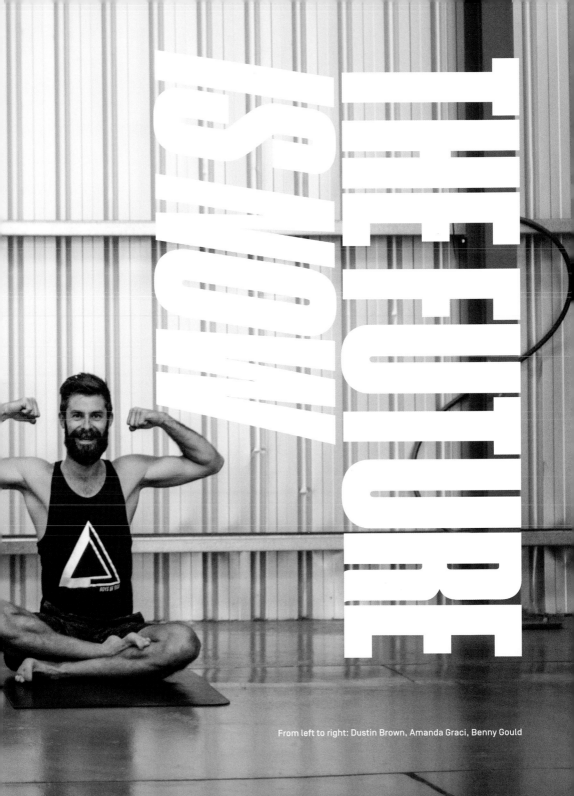

THE FUTURE IS NOW

From left to right: Dustin Brown, Amanda Graci, Benny Gould

If Not Now, When?

So that's it. The end of the book, but hopefully just the beginning of the conversation. My aim in writing this book was to share the practice of yoga from a different point of view: to celebrate and normalise men on the mat and living mindfully in the real world. Whether you're brand new to the practice or a seasoned sun-saluter; whether you're a guy thinking about taking your first class or a girl who's needed something like this to share with the guys in your life: whoever you are, wherever you are, I hope that this book will serve you or someone in your life and get them feeling confident enough to step onto the mat.

Throughout the pages of this book, and the many more stories, videos, classes and tutorials that can be found online at boysofyoga.com, it's always been about opening more conversations and creating a way for us all, boys and girls alike, to connect and see the value and benefit of a yoga practice. I hope you found something of value for your life and practice, wherever you are on your own personal yoga journey.

When I first started the project, people used to ask me what the long-term vision of BOYS OF YOGA was. And my answer was, to make the project pointless and entirely irrelevant. That may seem confusing or contradictory, but if we can shift the common conversation in the West so that people can see the real-world benefits of yoga, and if we can get an equal balance of men and women on the mat, then we no longer need to celebrate guys

in yoga. We've still got a lot of work to do, but if BOYS OF YOGA can help to get just one more guy on the mat and encourage him to step into a more mindful way of living, then it's been worth every moment of the journey.

So now it's the time to stop talking, and just try. Don't worry if you think you'll look ridiculous or you can't yet touch your toes – we've all been there. Trust me, the practice gets easier and the chaos will calm. So check your ego at the door and come inside. I guarantee you'll be glad you did.

If not now, when?

Find out more at **boysofyoga.com**
Join in the conversation at
@boysofyoga.com

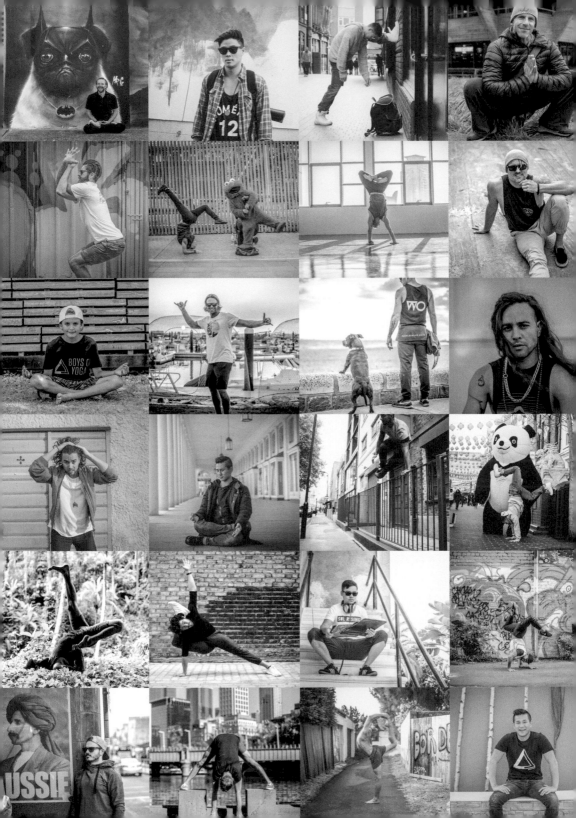

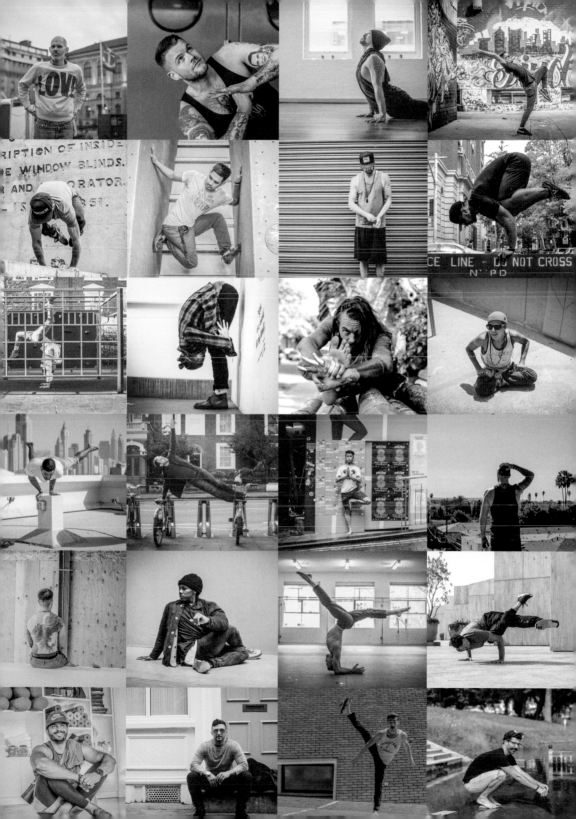

INDEX

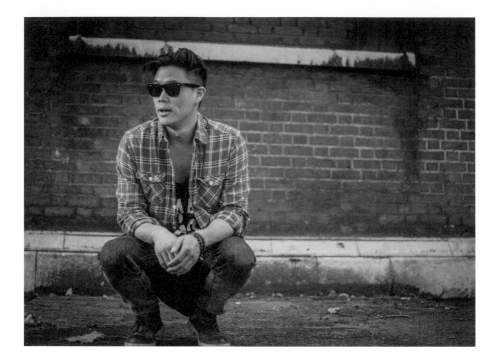

ABOUT THE AUTHOR

Michael James Wong is a Global Yogi and Wellness Warrior who is recognised around the world as a leading voice in the global wellness movement for yoga, meditation and modern mindfulness.

An inspirational speaker, international teacher, meditator and now author, Michael's passion is to inspire the masses about the benefits of a mindful way of living, on and off the yoga mat, every single day.

A Los Angeles native, now based in London, Michael travels the world sharing the benefits of the practice. Over the past 15 years he has been lucky enough to learn and study from some of the most inspiring teachers, spiritual leaders and global influencers around the world, all of whom have helped to shape his approach to modern mindfulness in the real world.

Founder and vision behind **BOYS OF YOGA**, Michael is a man on a mission to spread the word, break down barriers and stereotypes and bring the global wellness community together in a calmer and quieter conversation.

THANK YOUS

To my family who have been there every step of the way; Mom, Dad, Andrew and Nicole (and Erica, Max and baby Koa!).

To all the BOYS who have helped to bring this conversation to the world and to all my friends who have helped me, supported me, grounded me and inspired me.

To all my teachers, past and present, who have trusted me with their wisdom.

To Elena Brower for being you.

To Laura Gross and the Wanderlust family for giving me a chance.

To the HarperCollins team who worked tirelessly from day one to make this dream come true; Carolyn Thorne, Georgina Atsiaris, Ben Gardiner, Lucy Sykes-Thompson.

To my agent, Rachel Mills, and the Furniss Lawton team for helping me every step of the way.

To Whiskey Club and all the homies.

To our growing communities who inspire me daily; @boysofyoga, @justbreathelondon and @sundayschoolyoga.

And to Niki Priest, without whom this project would not have been possible.

Find out more about Michael at **michaeljameswong.com** or follow him **@michaeljameswong**
Find out more about the BOYS at **boysofyoga.com** or follow them **@boysofyoga**

Thorsons
An imprint of HarperCollinsPublishers
1 London Bridge Street
London SE1 9GF

www.harpercollins.co.uk

First published by HarperCollinsPublishers 2018

1 2 3 4 5 6 7 8 9 10

Text and Photography © Michael James Wong 2018
Photos on pages 15, 17 and 222 © Niki Priest 2018
Design Direction: Niki Priest

Michael James Wong asserts the moral right to be identified as the author of this work.

A catalogue record of this book is available from the British Library

ISBN 978-0-00-824965-6

Printed and bound in Latvia

The author and publishers of this work have made every effort to ensure that the information contained
here is as accurate and up-to-date as possible at the time of publication. However, it is recommended
that readers always consult a qualified medical specialist for individual advice. This book should not be
used as an alternative to specialist medical advice which should be sought before any action is taken. The
author and publishers cannot be held responsible for any errors and omissions that may be found in the
text, or any action that may be taken by a reader as a result of any reliance on the information contained
in the text which is taken entirely at the reader's own risk.

While every effort has been made to trace the owners of copyright material reproduced herein and secure
permissions, the publishers would like to apologise for any omissions and will be pleased to incorporate
missing acknowledgements in any future edition of this book.